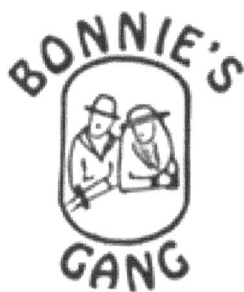

Bonnie's Gang Publishing is proud to present:

The seventh in a series of works for lovers.
Also by Jani:

Boink Her Pink
Got Milked?
BlowPons … Blowjob Coupons
G-gasm Method for Lesbian Lovers
Tonight's The Night
SexToysSell.com

Why Women Love
CAVEMEN

A MAN'S GUIDE TO TAMING THE BITCH

By: Jani Zubkovs - Published by Bonnie's Gang Publishing, New York

Although based on actual experience, some events in this book have been fictionalized to protect the privacy of certain individuals.

Please consult your Doctor if you are pregnant, have had a caesarean, surgery or infections before trying the Woman Tamed Sex Technique.

As with anything, use common sense.

Bonnie's Gang Publishing

http://BonniesGang.com

http://WomenTamed.com

ISBN: 0-9762090-9-8

FOR YOU, TO TAME THE WOMEN IN YOUR LIFE.

TABLE OF CONTENTS

FORWARD

As you well know, millions of men have essentially had their walnut sized stones wrenched out from under them … and have been sissified by the liberal media and the feminist movement.

I'm not talking about equality here – I'm all for that. I'm talking about pussifying men – making them sissies. Doing dishes or helping with the laundry or helping out with housework is NOT what "pussification" of men means--not by a long-shot. You can't "pussify" John Wayne by having him do a pile of laundry. Men and women can be equal without stripping away their fundamental roles.

I don't need to put down women or hold them as less than equal or submissive. Having "stones" has more to do with how to treat a woman --not put her down.

Liberal feminism's rise along with the entire "Politically Correct" movement has made it to where a guy can't be a guy anymore. We're taught to see ourselves as big, dumb providers. Need proof: Take a look at all the silly sitcoms on TV.

Young boys aren't just overly energetic and need to be engaged, they have ADD ---medicate them. We don't deal with that over exuberance as a natural thing, we try to "educate" that behavior out of the child.

You can go to a school or university and join women groups, go to colleges and attend classes on feminism. You can go into politics by exploiting feminism. Use feminism as a tool to advance almost any pet project you have. Not one of these things is possible for a male and I'm NOT saying there should be - there shouldn't be any of it – male or female.

Destruction of male group's pride and self worth is the norm in this "NEW" male world.

A new society is being constructed - one in which being a genuine and real man is becoming looked down upon. I see it here in America, Down Under, and it's very advanced in the UK and Europe.

This "sissification" of men is obvious in the media if you're aware of it. Keep an eye on ads on television; see if you can spot the subtle and not so subtle put downs of men. Usually, the husband is a dumb dolt and the smart wife has it all figured out. OR the woman is being a mature, responsible adult while the man acts like a child. It's a very irritating trend.

I describe a genuine man as being one who lives by honor, has the courage of his convictions who say what they mean and mean what they say, and who are fearless in their opposition to what they believe is wrong.

This sissification is evident everywhere.

So ...

How long have you been without your stones?

Are you purchasing tampons yet?

Time to put an end to the madness ... one woman at a time.

Time to man-up and start "Taming Your woman."

I DON'T WANT TO BE SEEENSIIIITIIIVE

Have you ever heard the phrase, "Men are from Mars, women are from Venus"? Men typically act in a very different way than women to the degree that people will often make interstellar metaphors as a way of showing the vast differences in the thought processes and behaviors between male and female.

Viva la Obvious!

Let's not make too much of an issue about the same thing you've heard time and time again from the enormous dung heap of romantic comedies that Hollywood feels obligated to rape our brains with each and every year. Most of these crappy movies have some metrosexual like Ben Affleck as the star. Being romantic at the right time and place is fine --- but I'm assuming, that by you reading this, you have a woman that needs taming – NOT romanticizing.

I won't bother with too much courtship bullshit and let's focus on the important stuff instead. This means that we will discuss the ways in which you'll need to change yourself and your woman if you truly want to have all that you need and want out of a relationship.

A woman is a lot like a lion. Lions have claws, they "roar" --- and according to the feminist doctrine you can "hear them roar", some of them live in Sub Saharan Africa, they playfully bite their children's necks and carry them around in their mouth, and…okay, well a woman is not exactly like a lion but a man who is looking for a woman is a bit like a lion tamer.

We don't carry the ubiquitous whips and stools but we do sometimes feel like we are about to be eaten alive if we don't do or act correctly (as far as she is concerned). Fortunately, taming a woman is not as difficult as taming a lion. In most cases, the only scars you will end up with will be on your heart, and you will be better for it.

IT ALL BEGINS WITH YOU

Have you ever heard of the saying, "To thine own self be true"? It may sound like the famous proverb but it really can carry some meaning when used in your personal life. Unless you truly know yourself, you can never know the world around you. This may be hard news for some of you to take but here it is: The reason why you may not be successful with women might have more to do with you than the women in question. Have you ever stopped to consider that your loneliness might be a result of your personality flaws and general "unlikability"? Why don't we delve into *that* Pandora's box for a minute, hmm? Let's consider the possibilities that may have led to your consistent failure with women in the past.

COMPASSION—Putting "com" in front of words can completely change their meaning. A "fort" for instance, brings to mind images of battle, fighting, and death. Add "com" to the front of it and you've got "comfort", a word that brings to mind peace, ease, and a general good feeling. Use the word "bat" and you have a violent weapon. Turn it onto "combat" and you have a bunch of guys hitting each other with bats.

The same rules apply when you hear women say they want a "passionate guy". A guy with passion is fine but make no mistake: Women want a passionate guy but a **COM**passionate guy is a **big no-no**.

Women always say they want to meet a nice guy but this is just to keep up appearances. Give a girl a nice guy and she'll shred him up faster than a lion shreds paper. This is because women don't want a doting and compassionate lover. Not often, at least. A too sensitive man triggers a "must cheat" command in the database of a woman's brain. Women like a good challenge. They like to be told what to do. They like dominance – especially during sex. More on all that later …

CLINGINESS: If you have a string of ex-girlfriends that only stuck around for a short period before leaving you, then please sit down while I tell you this. You, my friend, may be unlucky enough to be among the most despised and reviled groups of men to ever come along and send a shiver down the collective spine of the female sex. You might be a "clingy guy".

In the same way that women say they want a nice guy but actually desire much the opposite, women will say they want a guy who will always be there for her ready to do her bidding. Obviously, when this fantasy becomes a reality, it is not so pretty. A girl will soon find that a guy who constantly calls her and is madly in love with her after three dates is not the personification of the ideal man but more the archetype of a stalker who wears his lovers tampon around his neck bound with her used dental floss.

I call these people "hopeless romantics". This is because these people are hopeless when it comes to sustaining a lasting romantic relationship. They (maybe you included?) usually send out warning signals soon after the first date that scares the girls away.

Are you the "clingy" type? Let's take a look at some of the trademark behaviors associated with this unfortunate condition to see if you apply. If more than one of these apply to you, you may wish to rethink the way you approach relationships.

--You've discussed moving into her place before you've even eaten her pussy

--When you jack off you think about her instead of a hot porn star taking a giant cock up her ass while deep throating a midget.

--You can't wait to get the fucking out of the way so that you can get down with some awesome all-night cuddling and spooning with your sweetheart.

--Your "Y" chromosome is lower case

--The sonnets you write and leave on her car windshield are in iambic pentameter

--You write sonnets and leave them on her car windshield

You get the idea. Being a loving devoted man to

your sweetheart sounds like the ideal behavior of a man in love, but it can ruin your chances of steady pussy and a successful long-term relationship faster than Sammy Hagar ruined Van Halen. As much as you may not like it, you'll need a constant arm's distance from your woman in order to keep a challenge present. If you truly are in love with this gal, try not to let her know before you are sure that she feels the same way. This may go against every instinct in your heart, but you may have to treat her like a petty floozy.

MR. REMINISCENCE— Any girl will tell you that a guy, who still harbors feelings for his ex, instantly removes him from the guest list at Club Pussy. If you are one of the unfortunate broken-hearted suckers, for the love of God, don't tell potential ass about your feelings. Do what regular guys do: Drink her memory away in a river of whiskey and write rudimentary country songs about her, lamenting her loss. Lets look at the way such a situation plays out in the real world:

BILLY EVERYGUY: Wow, Jane. Thanks for suggesting this place. When I was going out with Beth, she always wanted to go to Olive Garden. Ugh, I HATE Olive Garden. Real, authentic Italian food my ass! I haven't been to Tuscany but I'll just bet their restaurants don't have a bunch of Dominicans cooking marinara in the kitchen and hitting on the fifteen-year-old hostess!

JANE PONTENTIALMATE: Uhh, no problem, Billy.

I heard this was the best place for biscuits in Averagetown.

BILLY: Ahh, Averagetown. I never knew how much nightlife there was. Fucking Beth always just wanted to rent movies from Blockbuster. Stupid Whore!

JANE: Do you still have a membership?

BILLY: You bet! I stole it from Beth when she left. It's a "Reward" membership. For every fifteen movies you rent, you get a free "old release".

JANE: Well why don't you go there and rent "How to lose a girl in ten minutes"?

BILLY: Okay, sure! Is it in the comedy section? Hey, where are you going?!

Billy missed what could have been the best sex of his life because he was still harping on Beth. Incidentally, "How to lose a girl in ten minutes" wasn't that bad. The theme was a bit heavy-handed but Diane Lane flashed her bush for a second. DYYYYEEE JOB!

Long story short, you have to be sure that, if you have hang-ups with your exes, you don't bring them up.

GBF (GAY BEST FRIEND) SYNDROME— In many cases, a guy will fall for a girl and make a fatal error: Instead of presenting himself as a sexual possibility, he will accidentally put himself in the position of becoming a friend. Think of Ducky from Pretty in Pink. If you find yourself in love with a woman, you must walk that thin line between friend and sexual interest. If you don't present yourself as a viable option for intercourse, you'll find yourself stricken with GBF syndrome.

You see, most women have what they call a "gay best friend". Some of these guys, maybe most of them, are gay. Many, however, are heterosexual guys who are hopelessly smitten, but have found themselves pigeonholed into a "friend" status. No matter what they do, they can't escape the stigma of a friend. Often, a guy like this is seen as a "brother" to the one girl who means the world to him. Have you ever been a Gay Best Friend unwillingly? Let's run through the list of symptoms:

-A girl you love or loved has confided in you about a guy she is interested in.

-You've been forced to listen to her sexual exploits with men she thought she liked before realizing they were total butt-holes.

-You've only been to platonic places like the mall and Panera Bread with a girl that you care about because you never had the balls to make a move.

-You are an artistic, unique, interesting guy who dresses funny intentionally as a way to set yourself apart from the crowd of sheep that worship the lady in question.

Often, the main reason why GBF syndrome comes about is an inability on your part to make a move. Let's take a look at the progression of your misery?

Once upon a time, you may have had a shot but you were too much of a pussy to go through with it. After a while, you lost any opportunity to become something to this woman. You might be saying to yourself, "This is all well and good, but how in God's name am I supposed to make a move? How am I supposed to show this woman that I'm, for lack of a better term, totally fuckable and hot?"

That's exactly where we'll begin. Let's face the facts; you may want to "tame a woman" for any number of reasons. Perhaps you're in love with a girl and you want her to feel the same passion that you do. Maybe you just want a bunch of steady ass. Either way, a large part has to do with fucking … namely, making her want to fuck you and keeping her wanting to fuck only you.

GET THE RIGHT ATTITUDE

Ok pay attention. I could write a whole book on this topic, there are extremely too many guys walking around with the wrong attitude. You are a man, so act like a man – be a man – don't be a girly-man.

You do not have to be debonair and sophisticated, you do not need any "moves," all you need is attitude - the right attitude, not the wrong attitude. There are ladies for all **men**, notice I emphasize men. Girls like: strong, weak, thin, husky – not fat, tall, short – well not too short, rugged, scrawny, young, old, you don't need perfect hair, perfect teeth, perfect skin, or a perfect body. In other words, unless you are a big fat disgusting slob with wind chimes dangling in your mouth disguised as teeth, there are girls out there for you.

Too many guys are walking around looking like they slept in a pile of dirty laundry. Groom yourself every day – shower, shave, trim your nose hairs and eyebrows, squeeze out those blackheads from your face, clip your nails and keep your hair clean and neat. When you are in a position to meet ladies – which is just about always – dress nice, and smell nice. Yeah, that's right, smell nice, put on some cologne – the ladies love that.

You need the right attitude. By attitude I mean your overall outlook and the manner in which you conduct yourself. Your feelings, your thoughts, the way you behave, your opinion of right and wrong and your way of thinking are all part of having the right attitude. Some attributes of the "right attitude," in no particular order of importance.

Smile a lot

Don't talk too much

Be a good listener

Be loyal to those that deserve your loyalty

Be clean and neat

Follow *your* traditions and values

Realize that getting there is 90% of the fun

Whatever you do – do it at 100%

It's **not** all about you

Be honest

Respect people that deserve respect

Try to help – especially when no one is looking

Be persistent

Dream – then plan

Are you going to do everything above all the time? No, but do get in the habit of having the right attitude, woman look for that in a man.

I am not a particularly good-looking guy; I'm about six feet tall and weigh 195 pounds. I have long light brown hair that is always clean and tied back in a ponytail. I have an acne-scarred face, that resembles the lunar surface, and when God was handing out noses, I thought he said roses – "I'll take the big red one in the corner," I said.

My usual attire is jeans, boots and some kind of a black tee shirt. I try to follow my own advice, and have the right attitude. I've never had a shortage of women, there were many times that I would be juggling 2 or 3 fuck buddies at a time. You know how that works - while you are banging one girl, you tell her that the other one is a pig. When you are banging the "pig," you tell her the other one is a slut.

WHAT WOMEN WANT (TO FUCK)

We should probably begin with a bit of the history of "attraction". Back in the caveman days, men were hunters and women were gatherers. You see this evolutionary throwback to this day in bars, where men are hunting for anything with two legs and three holes and women gather numbers they'll never call. At any rate, the continuation of our species depended on this give and take back in the day and we still see remnants of this everywhere we look.

You more than likely fall on one of the two major sides in this debate. Either you believe in true love and soul mates, or you believe that everything comes down to science and chemical attraction.

Eschewing the risk of leaving anybody out, let's assume that both sides are right. There are certainly biological factors that contribute to feelings of infatuation, but there are also such things as soul mates and true love. This way, we'll all be happy. Those that believe evolution is a myth still can't explain why there are dinosaur bones or fossils, when the world is only six thousand years old. Most atheists have good arguments for Darwin's theory but are at a loss when it comes explaining how everything started. Evolution explains the first organism, but it doesn't explain what caused that organism to become ALIVE. So, we're all right AND we're all wrong.

Let's get back to talking about the cavemen.

Back then, the human female needed a man who was physically strong. The man was a protector, defender and a necessary factor in the life of a female. In essence, everything back then depended on life and the continuation of it. Any second, a person could have been killed by a wayward mountain lion. That's why it was necessary to have a strong man who could, if not kill the mountain lion, at least keep him from snacking on the baby.

Admittedly, courtship was not as advanced as it is today. There were no sports bars for the cavemen to haunt and tell girls about their Firebird. There was only one club, and its use was to knock the woman out and drag her to the cave for a little R and R.

Don't think for a second that we've climbed much higher on the evolutionary ladder. Have you ever wondered why "beautiful" people are beautiful? Think of the stereotypical "sexy" man. He likely has broad shoulders, a V-shaped back, and a narrow waist. This build has appealed to women since before we had written language to pass notes back and forth.

But why are big shoulders and biceps sexy while large calves or big midsections aren't? They are all body parts, after all. The muscles in question indicated how fit and strong the man was. The more muscular he was, the more able he was to defend his mate and offspring. This is why women unknowingly swoon when they see the consistently shirtless Matthew McConaughey, although it might also have to do with his caveman brain structure, as well. Isn't it uncomfortable to know that, after thousands of years of evolution, our Cro-Magnon mindsets are still dominant in our brain?

Don't think men are any different, either. Why are men attracted to large breasts and wide hips? Why on earth would those specific parts of their bodies be more appealing to us than, say, the nape or the ankles? It is because large breasts and wide hips indicated to early man that the woman in question was better able to bear children and feed them. There it is, friends. There is the great mystery. Our basic ideas of attraction are only there to encourage us to subconsciously further our species.

So it is still true to this day: Women are more attracted to a man with a nice body. But that can't be all, can it? If we only look at the attraction between a man and a woman on a physical level, we run the risk of leaving out the one thing that unites humanity under one precept: Love. If it really is all just nature and biology encouraging us to mate, then there is no room for the poetic image of romantic love, is there?

I disagree with the idea that love, by itself, doesn't really exist and only has the importance that we as humans impose on it. All the same, it can be hard to stand steadfast to this dogma when there is so much evidence that we are simply animals with biological urges to mate that only seem important when they manifest in our minds as romantic ideas and concepts.

Ever heard of pheromones?

Pheromones are present in nearly all species of the animal kingdom. Pheromones are scents or odors emitted from the body whose intent is to cause a sexual desire in a member of the opposite sex. Sharks have them, vultures have them, and even skunks have them. The primate family (i.e. us) is no different. You may not know it but that deep attraction to that woman at the bar may have less to do with her slutty dress and more to do with a millennia-old primal urge unleashed because her glands are emitting "happy-stink". That's my term for pheromones and you can feel free to steal it.

This may remind you of those Axe and Tag body spray commercials where a guy sprays some product on himself and the females in the surrounding five-mile radius start coming (pun intended). The idea that certain scents can make the opposite sex more responsive to you is sound, if a bit exaggerated. Keep in mind that you aren't going to become an Adonis overnight by buying a five dollar spray can from the grocery store. If anything, those cheap scents are masking your natural odor that may be what actually makes you more attractive to the female.

While it can be very depressing to imagine that the concept of love and soul-mates are called into question by all of this science bs, remember that there is no scientific explanation for the reason that some people can finish each others sentences or why two people start to look alike after 30 plus years of marriage.

If you really want to "tame" this wild, pheromone-ridden, hunter-seeking beast, you'll need to grab her attention first. Most hunters are out for the kill. You're going to want to tame these women, but you may also wish to knock them dead with your sexiness. Deer hunters will sometimes rub copious amounts of deer piss all over them in order to attract deer. You won't be sneaking in the ladies room for a quick dab, but remember that the aim is to make them notice you. Once again, we'll have to look into the wild. Think of a peacock's feathers, or a lion's mane, or a lizard's big, gross, red thing that sticks out of his nasty throat. This attracts the females of their respective species. Don't think that humans are any different.

LET'S GO TAMEE HUNTING

Read the companion book in part two - "Element-X How to Meet, Date and Sleep with Killer Chicks" to discover the secrets of meeting and dating hot women. I'm not going into too much depth about meeting women at this point you can read all about that later. In a nutshell, Element-X is that thing that women refer to when they say "there's just something about him that I can't describe..."

Let's be honest with ourselves here. Unless you look like Orlando Bloom, you probably won't have too many women coming up to you. If you look like Orlando Bloom, you'll actually likely have a bunch of guys coming up to you as well. Either way, I'm going to guess you don't look like Orlando Bloom. You're still going to have to go up to a woman, more than likely, and basically sell yourself to her. Don't worry, though. We'll go through this mess together, and I'll set you up to look the part so you don't go in there looking like a moron. First, lets check out how well groomed you are.

You might think I'm going to tell you to shave your beard, lose the muttonchops, and ditch the lip piercing. Forget it. Remember how I said, "to thine own self be true"? Actually, I didn't come up with it. I think some English guy did. At any rate, keep that credo. You are you and there is no real way to change that. You can make that "you" more attractive to the opposite sex, but playing the part of someone else is eventually going to get your series cancelled.

That being said; keep the beard if you like it. Just don't get mad if you find that most women aren't into the Unabomber look. Keep the piercing, but don't expect to get a lot of attention from women who haven't heard of Sid Vicious. If you do decide that a change is needed, feel free! Your chin may not be as weak as you think. A shaved head might be better for your face. What I'm saying is, experiment if you want, stay the same if you'd like. Women are not as obsessed with looks as we guys are. Don't get me wrong; if you're ugly and you have huge, purple patches of scaling psoriasis all over your body … you're going to have a hard time no matter what, but that's not my problem. Take it up with God. As for those of you who don't look like Rocky Dennis (Mask), here are a few guidelines:

Women aren't necessarily anti-facial hair. They're more anti-Grizzly Adams. A bit of a shadow isn't bad and won't be seen as a deal-breaker. Some men look more attractive with a little fuzz. Others don't. Be your own judge. In times of war and economic troubles (like today, for example) men have traditionally been a bit shaggier, as a kind of statement on the situation of the world. You saw it in the 60's, and even in smaller recessions and high unemployment periods like in the '80s. Men's facial hair, as well as their hair in general, will usually be longer and women seem to respond to it more. There is a line, however. As far as goatees, soul patches, and other facial hair are concerned, it really comes down to you and your "try it and see if it works" attitude. Women on a whole, however, still frown on it. The more hair, generally, means the less likelihood of you bringing her home.

Mustaches with nothing underneath should be lost in nearly all cases. What do you want a mustache for anyways? You know they call them fanny-dusters, don't you? Do you think she wants a fanny-duster on her face? Cops wear them, for God's sake! So do perverts, Italian women and 70's porn stars!

While we're still on the subject of your face, let's take a look at those pores. Remember, they should resemble pores, not manhole covers. Having a clean mug can make more of a difference than you might think. Sure, you might say that women shouldn't be that shallow but maybe you should have thought about that before going to sleep without washing your face. Remember that your face will be the center of attention while talking to a girl that you intend to tame. You can bet that your chances of picking her up will dwindle as you talk to her and see her eyes furtively glance to that boil on your chin, unconsciously sneer, and then travel back up to your eyes. Try to keep your complexion smooth at all times and avoid going out to a bar if you aren't looking your best. Haven't you heard how important first impressions are?

Most men are clueless about dressing as well. While you don't want to be decked out in a three-piece suit if you are going to the local bar, you also can't expect success if you show up in a wife-beater and baggy jeans. Find a happy medium. Jeans are always in and they can instantly add to your appeal if you have a nice lower body. Remember that you are a man now and you can't wear baggy jeans that reveal your drawers. Don't go the emo route and wear skin tight jeans either. You want something that gives you breathing room but still hugs your ass and thighs enough to make yourself look somewhat fuckable.

Shoes are more important to women than most men ever care to find out. You don't need Italian loafers, but you certainly don't want to show up in white Reeboks covered in scuff marks. Tennis shoes overall are probably out, unless you are in a casual establishment that serves wings and domestic beer.

Cologne is another thing to keep in mind. While a dab here and there might help, remember not to overdo it or you'll smell like a Frenchman. In general, Frenchmen only get laid in France. Also be aware of the fact that, if you're a smoker, you are essentially wasting cologne if you use it. One cigarette may be all it takes to cover your clothes and skin in the stink of Parliament Lights.

Keep in mind that you don't have to necessarily be "attractive" if you want to get laid. If you recall earlier, when we discussed the caveman drives behind many of our emotions and attractions, you'll remember that women have this subconscious urge to mate with a man who is generally bigger, stronger, and tougher. This is why women like men to have big muscles and to do manly things. Scarred, rough, dry hands can make their soft, velvety vaginas wet.

While it might be discouraging to find that we may not have evolved as much as previously thought in the past few thousand years, we can still use this genetic predisposition to our advantage. While the Geico Cavemen will never be in People's list of the sexiest men alive, there are still aspects of our predecessors evident in many of us that can still make women swoon. You heard right: Some of your flaws that many consider repulsive may actually net you more women overall.

Most people would consider a unibrow to be the height of the bottom of the evolutionary ladder... or something like that. Truth be told, though, a unibrow can be seen as subconsciously attractive in the eyes of many a woman. The same goes for a big nose. For whatever reason, girls equate a large proboscis with a huge wang. A big nose is also seen as a mark of intelligence by some and, either way, big noses seem to have their own attraction factor and may stick in women's minds the way that sundial on your face sticks in the air.

A big forehead and even, god forbid, a sloping forehead can also impress connotations into women's minds of you being a burly, neanderthalian love-mongerer. Essentially, what the key point to focus in on is that you shouldn't be self-conscious about your flaws because they can be seen as attractive in the eyes of many women. Beauty, as they say, is in the eye of the beholder and you might find yourself some pretty sexy beholders that find your particular form of caveman chic downright appealing. You might even meet a nice girl named Lucy!

BE YOURSELF

Perhaps you're noticing that women don't really know exactly what they want. Prepare to have your mind further blown. Many of these things listed above that attract women sometimes fail wildly because of how many women are interested in the exact opposite.

Ever since Marlon Brando wore blue jeans and a t-shirt in some old-ass movie, women have swooned over the stereotypical image of the "Bad Boy". The Bad Boy is not a boy but, in fact, a man who generally does things that most would consider "bad". Of course, this is a sliding scale and is largely subjective. Dennis the Menace could be considered a bad boy, but so could Hannibal the Cannibal and Jack the Ripper. Colin Farrell is considered a bad boy because he smokes and swears in interviews, but Russell Crowe is a bad boy for beating people's heads in with telephones. There is definitely a line between bad boy and sociopath; between rebel and mass-murderer. The big question, though, is why would a woman go for a "bad boy", when it is clear from their description that they are, well, bad?

Many women will say that they went through a "bad boy" phase when they were younger. Often, the appeal of a bad boy to a teen girl is fueled by the disapproval of her parents. Any father would frown if his little girl brought home Chris Brown, and the catalyst for such an action can in fact have a lot to do with the need for attention. In the same way that strippers get naked for money because Daddy didn't love them, many girls like bad boys because the danger factor gets them attention that they otherwise may have been lacking.

This isn't to say that bad boys and rebels aren't attractive to many girls. Plenty of females have that nurturing instinct about them that can sometimes be over-applied in certain instances. Some women may find themselves consciously or subconsciously falling for or going after shady guys because there is a part of them that wants to "change" that guy; to "save" him.

Did I mention that women are insane?

In essence, "Bad Boy", as retarded as it sounds and as painful as it is to say, is not just a term, it's a way of life. Dressing like a thug or being rude in public doesn't necessarily make you a bad boy. It might just make you a prick or a big asshole.

Plenty of decent guys might accidentally fall under the umbrella term of "bad boy" just based on their actions. For instance, a generally "good guy" might have a drug problem and so may be called a "bad boy" despite evidence otherwise. A guy might be a reformed criminal but may still keep his "bad boy" status. In short, the term is too broad and convoluted to have any real meaning. Basically, it can be summed up with another adage equally as old. "Women fall for jerks". This keeps the same general idea while making it not so much about the guy, because it isn't, but about the girl.

Women fall for jerks because women sometimes need them. There is a short time in your life where you can be a "bad boy" or a "jerk" and have women fall for you. Once you hit forty or so, you'll be seen less as a sexy rebel and more as a dumb asshole.

Perhaps you aren't a bad boy and you are instead the opposite. You might be a nerd, dork, dweeb, geek, loser, douche, dildo, twerp, spaz, or any other application given to a guy who is generally smart and responsible. If you are a "nerd", you should rejoice. You, my friend, are living in the Age of the Nerd. You're a god in this day and age. Act like one!

Gone are the stereotypical ideas of nerds being shoved in lockers and getting sand kicked in their face by bullies who whisk away their girls. These days, people know that the nerds are the future rulers of the world. Nobody wants to screw with a nerd anymore, especially not in school. They'll either be your boss in two years or shoot you in the face in two weeks.

Finally, women are seeing that these people are not bespectacled, awkward goons who can't please them sexually. These people are in fact powerful, wealthy, brainy guys who can keep their ladies happy and satisfied far longer than some dumb all star quarterback who ends up hawking vacuum cleaners door to door and gaining seventy pounds on his midsection.

You need to embrace whatever kind of person you are. If you're a nerd, don't try to be a bad boy. A real bad boy will just remove your teeth for you. Be happy that you're intelligent and able to master things that the rest of us grunt at. Women are insanely attracted to guys who are able to use their brains for more than just thinking about pussy.

Again, like I said earlier, let's not spend too much time talking about picking up women, however. For that, read the accompanying book called "Element-X". Element-X goes into detail on how to meet, date and sleep with hot women.

You are more than likely at the point where you have a woman or almost have a woman, and you just want to make her yours. You want to "tame" her. Let's assume that she's already interested and now you just need to make her your "tamee". With that in mind, why don't we set to working on not only "taming" this girl domestically (i.e. so she is not constantly breaking your chops about doing man things like drinking beer, hanging with the guys or golfing) but more importantly sexually (it's amazing how little problems in a relationship disappear when the sex is great).

MEN AND WOMEN ARE DIFFERENT (NO SHIT!)

You ARE supposed to notice the major differences between men and women in regards to falling in love. Men, as you well know, are very fond of porn, strippers, frat parties, and any other situation that leads to girls being naked and showing you their various holes and boobs. This is because men are wired to feel a deeper attraction to the visual aspects of sexuality. Hence I've come to the conclusion that, "men fall in love through the eyes, but woman through their ears".

This is precisely why women spend so much time primping and making themselves beautiful before they go out, and why the makeup, skin care, hair, and clothing industries pull billions apiece easily every year. Women know how shallow and stupid we are when it comes to relationship building, but they acknowledge that it isn't our fault. Some of us men may be better and superior lovers than other men, but a woman will have to garner our attention the same way no matter who we are. Granted, a beautiful girl is still beautiful in sweatpants and sans makeup, but we may not notice it. We're looking at life in a different light then women are, let's admit it.

Many women are shallow, just like us, but they aren't turned on and off so easily and with such ease as us men are.

Think about the reason why women don't particularly care for porn (though many women do), and then look at the vast popularity of romance novels. It would almost seem that women would rather HEAR about hot, sexy, action rather than seeing it.

Take for instance the consistent popularity of the romance genre: 32 percent of adult mass-market paperback sales are romances, and Harlequin is the dominant publisher of hot-body stories worldwide. In 2008, it sold more than 130 million books; since its inception sixty years ago, Harlequin has shipped more than 5.7 billion books.

According to Harlequin, more than half of their readers have some college education and almost 50% work a full-time job. So it's not all just women cleaning their toaster in a house dress dreaming about escaping with Mr. Right. Romance readers are real, everyday women.

So that's what it come down to: romance for women and pornography for men. Male fantasies are rather adolescent in nature, but the underlying premise remains the same --- wild sex without responsibility. For women sex meaningful and symbolizes a lasting emotional connection, and often an end to financial responsibilities and money worries.

Many Harlequin stories have a scene where the heroine is 'broken in or tamed,' both emotionally and physically, by the male character. This is what makes romantic fiction attractive to women — the sexual and mental submission of women to men. Most women won't admit it, but this male mastery is what appeals to them. If it didn't, there would not be almost 6 billion books sold and shipped with that premise.

Consider this when talking to your woman: Sure, she may be attracted to you, but she may not act on it until you talk to her and she "reads" what you have to say. Women soak their seats over good dialogue! Tell her the right things, tell her what she wants to hear, and you had better believe that you will be on your way to taming her.

Think about it: When you see all these beautiful, GORGEOUS women walking around with these ugly, douchey guys, what do you think allowed this man to be fucking supreme tail in that princess/caveman relationship? Besides, him maybe having a huge cock, it is likely that he tells her all the right things and acts like a man.

WHAT WOMEN WANT (TO HEAR)

So it is clear, that you will have to talk a big game to do the big tame (where do you think the term 'game' came from in regards to talking girls into fucking?). If you want to get your "tame" on, start talking. So what do you say? I'm not talking about crappy pick-up lines in a bar, or any of that shit. I'm assuming you're already in earshot of ass, and you just need that final thrust to get into foreign territory.

Women love to hear about how beautiful they are, but the problem is that beautiful women have heard the same shit from every guy since they started bleeding from their snizz. Don't say "baby you look so hot" or "Damn you got some nice-ass tit-tays" because they've been hearing that same shit for years. Besides, it's pretty crude anyways. What's wrong with you? Didn't you ever learn how to respect women, you fucking troglodyte!?

Try complementing them on what they REALLY want to be complimented on. If you see them spending an hour with a straightening iron, don't tell them they look fine as hell. Tell them that their hair looks beautiful straightened, even though you loved it before they put the iron to it. Something like that should really get them slippery down there. Essentially, you want to use your fucking brain before you open your mouth.

Think about all the time that women spend trying to look pretty. If you take notice of these things, and believe me when I say it is not difficult, it is only a simple matter of pointing out the obvious. Tell her that her dress is beautiful. She likely hasn't heard that one before, at least not from a straight male.

Try complementing them on things that nobody notices. Women are insane when it comes to shoes. Tell her that you like her heels. Say they make her look even more beautiful. When it comes to complementing her on her body, tell her how beautiful her teeth are, or how lovely her calves are shaped. It may sound weird and you could run the risk of coming off as a fetishist but, if done right, you can score some major points. You can assume that, if she has pretty eyes, she's been told her entire life how beautiful she is. Try to set yourself apart from these morons! Using the same lines that countless guys before have dropped is like trying to get to Davenport by using a map from the 1920s.

With all of this talk about talk, let's not forget the one thing that ranks above nearly everything else when it comes to what women are attracted to: A sense of humor. A guy that can make a woman laugh can essentially hold her in the palm of his hand. Don't believe me? Jim Carrey is fucking Jenny McCarthy. Dane Cook fucked Jessica Simpson. Seal is fucking Heidi Klum (okay, he just LOOKS funny).

If you can make a girl laugh, you have a sizable lead on the competition. Most guys are morons and will talk about how awesome they are and how much money they make. Don't get me wrong, girls like confidence and bravado, and they also like money quite a lot. The problem, though, is that you often come across as an arrogant cocksucker. Being funny can assuage that problem, and self-deprecating humor can even be a turn-on to many girls. Being able to laugh at yourself shows its own kind of confidence.

If you are naturally a funny guy, use that god-given talent to your advantage. In all probability, you have already seen how attractive humor is to a girl and have bedded girls way out of your league simply because you made them smile and laugh. Like we've been discussing, the quickest way to a woman's heart is through her ears.

In addition, you must understand that being funny ALL of the time can be just as detrimental to your purposes as being dryer than an 80-year-old woman's pussy all the time. Being too goofy, fun, and fancy-free can make you resemble a Disney character more than a man. If you are too wacky, zany, nutty, or silly, you can joke your way right out of a relationship.

Outwardly, most women have no idea what they want. They are attracted to a guy who is funny, but if he isn't serious when he needs to be, he's cut off. They want a guy to be sweet and caring, but if he comes off as a pushover, he's excommunicated. Being confident is a necessity in taming a woman, but being overly arrogant can get you on the B or even C list. With that in mind, lets look at the crazy and intimidating world of confidence!

CONFIDENCE vs. ARROGANCE

By now, you've probably picked up on how big a role evolution and biology play in our mating habits and preferences. Pretty sad, huh? Well, if you want to tame a woman, you're going to have to get into the mind of the tamee … she LOVES confidence.

Webster's Dictionary defines confidence as being sure of yourself. This character trait appeals to women because it evokes in their mind the image of the bold, Cro-Magnon tough guy. The problem, though, is that you need to strike the right chord between arrogance and -- well "pussiness" – for lack of a real word. Webster's Dictionary defines "pussiness" as being really into Barry Manilow. All joking aside, you must be able to strike a harmonious chord between being arrogant and being confident. Let's take a look at the differences:

An arrogant guy lets everybody know how awesome he is. He'll be the first to espouse the virtues of how great he is. A confident guy, on the other hand, shows his awesomeness not by his speech, but by his actions. If he's the best at something, he'll be the last to tell you about it. The confident man helps someone when no one is looking. An arrogant man only helps someone when he helps himself.

An arrogant guy controls his woman in front of other people because he wants to show how dominant he is. A confident guy knows that he has the upper hand and has no need to show off to other people the level of control he has.

Are you getting the picture? Women love confidence. Newton once said that for every action, there is an equal and opposite reaction. Newton probably got a whole lot of pussy. His lessons live on. If women love confidence, then women despise and detest the opposite of confidence, which is insecurity. Insecure guys are pussy kryptonite. Why is this so? Because insecurity evokes the idea that you need to be taken care of and you need to be babied. This makes you seem like a woman, and the only women who like other women aren't going to like you unless you get a sex change. Here's how you can avoid appearing insecure, even if you are.

Don't bitch: There are some things that are worth raising a fuss about, but there is a difference between addressing a problem assertively and complaining about shit like a teenage girl. Don't ever throw a fit. "Fits" automatically relegate you back to a sexual non-interest. Showing that you can handle any problem with tact and reason shows that you are a strong male who is able to hold his demeanor no matter what comes your way. That shows confidence, wouldn't you say? Say it out-loud!

 Do bitch: There are times when it is necessary for you to show your mate that you can solve problems. In the caveman days, the females did not look kindly at the men who couldn't make a fire, or keep them dry in the rain. These girly-guys were forced to a cave to work on drawings on rock walls. If there is a problem with the service in the restaurant where the two of you are dining, take care of it. Don't sit there and wait for the problem to resolve itself. If someone cuts in line at the club, if someone is playing their music too loud too late, you should be able to deal with the problem. Solving problems shows that you are both confident enough to address an issue and mature enough to diplomatically avoid an altercation and man enough to punch somebody in the nose if it comes to that. Try and talk your way through things, but if push comes to shove ... Get it?

Jealousy: This one is a bit tricky. You can't go flying off the handle every time that she talks to a guy on the phone or makes eye contact with someone at the mall. You can't be too suspicious and inquisitive when she is out with her friends. That will make you seem possessive and insecure about your hold on her.

On the other hand, if you play it too cool and act too confident, she will think you could care less about what she does and who she's with. You need to strike a happy medium where you express slight jealousy when appropriate so that she knows you want her and that you acknowledge her beauty and attractiveness to the opposite sex. You can't be too controlling, though, or she will think you have an inferiority complex, which is the antithesis of confidence.

In time, you'll learn to tell the difference between what is too passive and what is too aggressive. Most men simply don't have the confidence to even approach a beautiful woman they are attracted to, let alone pull off a taming and proceed to seduce her.

Being nervous, scared and weak is NOT

something most women (especially hot ones, ready to be tamed) find sexy and attractive in a man – it's actually a big turn-off. Being confident, comfortable, fearless and in control is something most women find extremely attractive. Remember that confidence begins with you.

Are you confident? If not, get self-confident and positive. Start with the simple easy to use guide you received with this book – "Caveman Secrets to Sexual Power."

"Caveman Secrets" is a five step plan:

Eat right and eat raw.
Drink pure water.
Exercise five times per week.
Get plenty of sleep.
Walk every day.

Go to Part III foe more detail.

It sounds easy, because it is. This is not rocket science.

Your girl obviously sees something in you if she's with you, so use that as your lighthouse when you start to drift among the seas of self-doubt.

Remember that you're trying to tame a woman. Approaching everything with a confident demeanor is the way to go if you want the result to involve her. But with so many problems that can come along, how can you keep your cool and maintain composure? Well, let's take a look at the various factors that can sour a relationship and keep you from taming your quarry. Or is it prey? Let's just move on and leave the genus phylum shit to the taxidermists?

TAMEE BAGGAGE

Taming a woman is hard enough work as it is. What makes it more difficult, however, is dealing with a woman who has baggage from her childhood. Daddy issues, control problems, all types of matters can lead to shock and awe in the mind of a man who thought, for once, that he had actually met a normal woman. Let me tell you right now, no woman is normal. No woman is completely sane. To be fair, no man is sane either. It all comes down to childhood and upbringing.

Some women have what psychologists refer to as "daddy issues". Daddy issues can spell doom for even the most compatible couple, that is, unless the man in the relationship is willing to either play along with the sick charade or snap the girl out of it. Either way, you have to keep your eyes peeled for warning signs of daddy issues. To better prepare you, lets take a slightly more in-depth look at daddy issues.

Remember when Norman Bates said that a boy's best friend is his mother? Well, in the same way that many men who are psychotic or violent have unhealthy relationships with their mothers, the problems of many women trace back to her father. For the most part, a father/daughter relationship is typically healthy and the girl is "daddy's little princess". But what if the daddy wasn't nice enough to the girl? What if daddy touched her? With his penis? A girl who wasn't properly loved by her dad will often grow up into a girl who subconsciously tries to get back at daddy. Many girls who are strippers, porn stars, or otherwise take dick for money have an unhealthy or no relationship with their father.

This isn't the only way that daddy issues can manifest themselves, however. A girl with a mean or abusive dad will often be more sexually explicit and hornier than the average girl, but a girl who had a dad who wasn't around or who largely ignored her has daddy issues of a completely different, and arguably more disturbing kind.

Sigmund Freud was many things, a psychologist, German, pervert (I'm sure), and genius. He caught a lot of dissension in the 1920's for changing the way we look at our minds by associating almost everything from bananas to dreams with sex. Freud often spoke about how our formative years with our parents shape us for the rest of our lives.

Later on, many psychologists disagreed with Freud and lay to rest some of his claims, but there is still a sizable body of evidence that our parents, for better or worse, shape what is to be our adult lives.

Think about the preceding few paragraphs, talking about how girls become whores to get back at their daddies. Obviously there are exceptions that prove the rule, but it is staggering how many sluts have daddy issues.

This is often because of abuse on the part of the father.

But what if your girl's daddy didn't necessarily physically abuse his daughter? What if he simply neglected her or mentally abused her? This situation sets the foundation for the daddy issue we're talking about now.

Instead of a girl trying to get back at her dad by being a slut, many girls who seem perfectly normal engage in relationships wherein they try to REPLACE their daddy. Whether you like it or not, your sweetheart may only be interested in you because she sees a flash of her daddy in you: The daddy who didn't pay attention to her, or the dad that never went to her class play. This may seem weird and maybe a little hot, but it can turn into disaster down the road.

Maybe you look like her daddy. Maybe you talk and act like her daddy. Maybe she didn't know her daddy too well and every boyfriend she's ever had has been, to her, a surrogate daddy. Either way you slice it, it is generally a kind of fucked-up situation. Sure, you will almost certainly have the upper hand in the relationship, and she will more than likely be submissive to you, but you may also have to deal with some repressed emotions that you didn't ask for.

In many of these cases, the relationship is marred beyond repair because the girl will pout, whine, and otherwise act like a child in order to get her way. Sometimes she will do it just for attention. As opposed to a healthy relationship, where this preferably wouldn't happen, you are in a sick, incestual, relationship where your sweetheart is trying to use you as a replacement father figure. Can't you just see the repercussions?

Are you playing daddy and don't even know it? Let's take a look at two major warning signs:

-You bear a casual or striking resemblance to her father when you look at pictures of her family

-Your girlfriend constantly pouts, whines, and complains until she gets her way, or otherwise becomes a child when you're around despite the fact that she acts normal and mature in public and at work.

Do any of these apply to you … if so, it isn't the end of the world.

We've covered the two main types of daddy issues that you need to understand in order to get this woman under control. These types of women are actually very easy to tame. Besides the sexual aspect of taming, which we get into detail later, keep reminding her in subtle ways that you are the new "dad." A reprimand there, a scowl when something is not done to your satisfaction, a frown on your face when she says something you deem inappropriate. She'll get visions of dad in her head and quickly be as tame as a bunny rabbit.

Now that I've called your girlfriend a disgusting slut and an incestual monster, let's move on to more innocuous manifestations of baggage. You may not like it, but we're going to have to talk about your lover's former lovers. Shudder now and get it over with.

GHOSTS OF BOYFRIENDS PAST

Every woman has an ex or two or three. Perhaps this is why many men go for younger women ... I DON'T mean between ten and twelve. You might not be able to match up to the many men who have been inside the heart and pussy of women your age, but you can certainly show an eighteen-year-old a better time than Billy Boy down the road can. His idea of a passionate night is a 2 liter of Mountain Dew and a Suite Life of Zach and Cody DVD. What a douche ...

Many girls have hang-ups because of guys they used to date. Actually, ALL girls have issues because of past relationships. It is just a matter of scale. This can be a disastrous roadblock in your path to taming a woman, and you have to act accordingly.

Often, a woman will be unable to trust you because a man in her past was totally unfaithful and dishonest to her. That cocksucker pretty much fucked you over, because now you have a suspicious and distrusting woman on your hands. She will go through your call log on your cell phone, call you at odd hours to make sure you're where you say you are, and plotting the murder of your ex-girlfriend that calls you here and there. You explain to her that the ex and you are just really good friends now and there's nothing going on even though you were over at her house two weeks ago and didn't think it was worth mentioning until it came to light. Why was there a Timberlake CD in your car? You don't like Timberlake. Whose CD was it?

Having to constantly reassure a girl that you're faithful, may be a sign that she has ex baggage. She probably had an ex that cheated on her. You have to assume control of this woman and you need to tame her into a more docile creature. But how does one go about this? Well, you need to reassure your girlfriend that you are faithful and she has nothing to worry about because you aren't about to go out and get it on with some cheap floozy because you care about her: She's the one.

If you can't convince your honey that you only have eyes for her, let her know that her insecurities regarding you are based on her inability to get over her trust issues that were given to her as a result of the unfaithfulness of one of her former lovers. These thoughts will either give her the chance to do a bit of self-reflection and soul searching, or it will confuse her enough to get her off your back for a second.

You might have to look at the world through her eyes for a moment. It may be rather annoying when her eyes are constantly looking at your Email inbox, but you must remember that it isn't her fault. Not totally, at least. Work through these latent trust issues together to soften and let you in her now rock-hard heart. Then you can cheat on her all you want ;)

Sometimes the problem isn't one of trust but one

of longing. Specifically, the girl may still be harboring some feelings for one of her exes. This is a losing battle my friend. A girl who still clings to the love of the past may as well be made of stone. That doesn't mean you can't stick your sword in the stone, but it certainly won't feel very comfortable, will it? As pitiful as a guy can be when getting over an ex, girls can be even worse in these situations. This is because of those wacky hormones and emotions that girls get.

If you are dealing with a woman who is still in love with her former lover, you might just want to get the fuck out of Dodge. Trying to get a woman to move on when she isn't ready is a real uphill battle, with a landslide as your enemy. This doesn't mean that you can't FUCK her though. Hear me out for a sec, will ya?

Sure, you may not be able to sustain a relationship with a girl who is still all hung up on one of her exes, but you may be able to use that longing to your advantage. Try to learn all you can about her ex, and you may be able to act as a sexual substitute.

Like we've been discussing, women are completely crazy and they may use you as a means to achieve a certain end. Normally, this would be considered offensive to a guy, but if you are getting pussy as well as mentally manipulating a lonely girl who only craves the love she will never have again, who is the real winner?

Don't get me wrong, this is scandalous and, well, wrong, but don't you think it's kind of screwed up for a girl to fuck a guy just because he reminds her of her ex? We've all been the pitcher, and we've all been the catcher … and sometimes we all hate the game.

Suppose the problem isn't the memory of an ex so much as the physical presence of kids. This is a different situation. Often, if you are fooling around with a woman who has kids, you may have to deal with the father of said children. You can't very well ask your woman to keep him out of her life … he's the pater familias. In these situations, you will have to maintain a somewhat decent relationship with the dude, no matter how tenuous it may be. Just hope that the guy can't kick your ass, am I right? Don't be his bitch, but try to see where he is coming from. You're fucking the mommy of his little ones!

Now is a good time to also look at the "Spoiled Brat Factor". Rare is the roadblock in the relationship that is as immense and detrimental as this little problem. Let's not sugarcoat the facts: Some (a lot of) women are spoiled little bitches, or maybe not even spoiled, but bitches at any rate. Sometimes it is because they were and sometimes still are, treated like a princess by their daddy. Often, it is because they ran through a slew of boyfriends who they walked all over. In many cases, it is a combination of both.

Whatever way you slice it, the vast majorities of

these women are hot physically, but take a lot of taming to get them where they should be. Being "hot" is why they have been spoiled so much. Hot girls always get what they want. They never have to pay for their drinks, they can get any guy they want, and there is always some poor sap willing to trade a few bucks and a couple dollops of pride in exchange for pussy. Hmm, maybe he's not such a sap after all … He will definitely end up poor, though. That is, if she sticks around long enough to dry up his resources.

That's not happening to you.

I have a good friend named Mike. Mike 's a nice guy, married to Gloria for the past seven years, they have a couple of little kids and a house in the suburbs.

Mike is a Cro Magnum man at work. He's a tough guy, runs a small construction company with four employees and never takes any shit from customers, employees, subcontractors or suppliers.

Mike makes a very good living, but there is one thing he does every two weeks that drives me crazy. He hands his paycheck to Gloria.

Don't ever let me catch you handing your paycheck to your tamee.

Money is power. Look around the real world. Those people that control blocks of cash wield power. On a smaller scale, the one in a relationship that controls the finances commands the respect of those that don't. Seize control of the checkbook and all financial accounts and dealings.

You see, spoiled little bitch girls are like parasites. You give them what they want until you have nothing left to give. Then they get rid of you like a bad case of crabs. Hey, wait a minute….who was the parasite again …

Because a girl is a spoiled bitch, doesn't mean you have to bend over backwards or bow to her whims. That is just what she wants you to do.

Or is it?

No, it isn't.

She is longing and begging for taming. She doesn't want to be a spoiled snotty little bitch -- she wants to get off that roller coaster ride of abusing men that sit there and take it up the ass like little sissy-men. TAME her, be dominant, and her snootiness' disappears. Girls like a CHALLENGE. This is why the GBF and the "nice" guy fail so spectacularly all the time.

DON'T give her what she wants, and what she wants will become YOU.

If you haven't noticed by now, the key idea is for you to maintain the upper hand no matter how difficult it may seem at times. If you recall, we touched a bit on the things that turn women off. Most of them have to do with weakness on the part of the male. Obviously, it should go without saying that the opposite of weakness and indecision in a man should fill women with feelings of attraction and lust.

You need to learn the art of "domination". This doesn't mean that you should buy whips and chains. We're focusing on the mental aspects of domination right now. Don't worry, we'll talk about the physical part – "how to tame her through sex" in a few minutes.

DOMINATION: MAINTAIN THE UPPER HAND

If this book gets into the hands of any females, I'm in deep shit.

Domination is a big bag of worms to get into, but let's focus on the basics first. We all know that most women, whether up front or deep down, like, need, and desire domination.

How much is relative, but women respond better to a man who takes charge. There is nothing less sexually appealing to a female than a man who is wishy washy, weak, or can't make decisions. It is the sign of a, well, a pussy. Girls hate pussies, even though they have them. Perhaps it is because they have them, that they don't want a life-sized one to haul around and stand there while they make all the decisions.

There is, of course, the opposite risk. You don't want to be TOO domineering or you'll choke the plant that is your love with the smoke that is your desire for control. Women are a funny breed. Most women like domination from their mate because it feels right, you can't shrug off thousands of years of evolution in an instant. The key thing, though, is to make sure that you walk that fine line from being dominating to being domineering.

Women around the world will tell you how much they hate an indecisive man. Keep your tentative, weak voice in check or you'll be spending a lot of time alone at night spanking your monkey. This is a "must do". If you can't take the reins and make some decisions, you might as well call it a night.

When meeting a girl for the first time, it all starts with your handshake greeting. You being wimpy with your handshake, right off the bat sets off her "pussy radar." Give her a hand a nice solid squeeze --- not too hard, but don't just grab her fingertips. Make sure you give a deep, firm, thumb to thumb handshake.

Try to take control when planning a date. Don't ask the girl what she wants to do because it can have disastrous effects the likes of which you haven't seen since you first walked in on your mom in bed with your dad.

 If you ask the girl what she wants to do, and she says she doesn't know and lobs the question back to you, you'd better have something to add. Don't say you're fine with anything, and don't say that you want to do whatever she wants to do. Women equate this mindset with weakness in a man, and you can bet that no woman wants to be laying under a chick with a dick. Well, maybe some women like it. If this is the case, I recommend you don't bring up the idea of strapons and pegging (unless you are into that).

Take the initiative and plan the date. Tell her what you're going to do. If the woman starts calling the shots, you'll quickly find yourself in the Gay Best Friend bracket or worse yet … divorce court. Lots of luck, Ducky!

Again, remember that there is a line. Be in charge as much as you can, but exercise a little prudence when necessary. You don't have to order for the girl. This is a touchy area and most women typically find it insulting if a man chooses her meal and orders it for her. Sure, this is an example of what a dominating man might do and, in theory, girls should like those ideas, but girls, as we all know, are fucking loony. Don't tread on their rights. They want to be dominated, but they don't want to be treated like a child or a moron.

Remember in Spinal Tap when they said that there was a fine line between stupid and clever? Well the line between being lovingly authoritarian and being a jerk or a dominating boyfriend and a bully is equally thin. Be careful when walking that line – never be a jerk or a bully.

SEX AND THE TAMEE

Before we get to the bedroom aspect of taming your woman there are a few things we need to discuss. Sex domination can turn your woman into the lady you truly want. Sex is a very powerful human drive and emotion. Some well-known philosophers and famous authors speculate that sex is the driving force in most things that we as humans do.

The great Napoleon Hill said, "Sex desire is the most powerful of human desires. When driven by this desire, men develop keenness of imagination, courage, will-power, persistence, and creative ability unknown to them at other times. So strong and impelling is the desire for sexual contact that men freely run the risk of life and reputation to indulge it."

Sex and sexual drive is both powerful and intoxicating. Instead of abusing that power, you need to discover how to harness the power of sex. Don't ever force sex or rape her. This should be self-explanatory but you'd be surprised how many guys think rape of a girlfriend or wife is no big deal. It is a big deal.

Remember that the bedroom is, essentially, the war room when it comes to relationships. What you do in the sack can be seen as a microcosm of your entire relationship with this tamee. If you are soft, weak, and generally pussy-esque, you will more than likely be on the bottom, and essentially be a dick with a body attached.

If you are TOO overbearing and TOO domineering, sex will probably involve the girl being bent over and spreading her ass cheeks. She will probably not enjoy it as much as if you were a little more levelheaded, and you probably get off quick while she doesn't get off at all. Sure, you showed her who is the boss but what satisfaction does she (or you) get out of it? You have to pay attention to her, Brutus! If she doesn't get satisfied by you … she'll be swallowing somebody else's load.

In a few minutes, you'll see how to dominate her by giving her orgasms --- almost at will. That is the power of the Women Tamed Technique (WT Technique).

The question you probably are asking is: "How am I supposed to be dominant and aggressive but not come off as a bully? How can I be sweet and nurturing while still keeping her interested?"

It is a rather difficult trick to pull off, but you can tame your woman by being a dominant male figure and still be sweet, nurturing and loving. Like we've discussed earlier, too much niceness can spell doom, but too little niceness will have much the same result. We'll have to find that happy medium wherein you can be a controlling, dominating lover, like she craves, while still being the tender and nurturing sweetheart, like she desires. First, let's sweeten you up:

YOUR SWEET SIDE

Thus far, we've spent very little time discussing the importance of being nice and kind. If anything, we've mostly been deriding guys who are tender and nurturing. You might take this as a cue that any sensitivity on your part is a death sentence for a relationship, but women DO need T.L.C., even though it can be a huge turn-off to them.

Though it seems paradoxical and counter-intuitive to be doting and loving on occasion, it should be pointed out that guys who are super sweet and cuddly only fail because they are ALWAYS like that. Girls like a challenge. Remember back pages ago to when we were talking about clingy guys. Sure, there is nothing wrong with being madly in love with a girl you just met, but if you let her find that out, she is instantly less attracted to you. The game is tarnished. It's too easy now. Why should she put forth the effort when you are already licking her stiletto heels? She would rather be with a guy who puts up a little resistance.

But what if you put up nothing but resistance? What if you took control, but never let her voice heard? Surely, this will get old just as the guy who is always sweet would eventually kill her with diabetes. Think of a relationship like a food or a drug: Everything in moderation. Too much sweetness is killer; too much harshness is killer. Fuck, if you eat too much nutmeg you'll die (if you eat just enough you can trip), a little on your pancakes or French toast (tamee cooks the majority of the time) is delicious. You need to strike the right chord in order to be exactly what this woman wants. But how can we be sweet and caring without running the risk of becoming THAT girly-guy? Well, a few maneuvers if you pull them off right, can allow you to be Mister Perfect.

CONVERSATION IS KING

Remember the phrase, "Men fall in love through the eyes, but woman through their ears".

Let's look at the way you talk to this potential tamee. I don't mean pick-up lines or anything like that. I mean regular, everyday conversation and "pillow talk". We are assuming that you already have the means with which to enter this woman coitally, but you are in the process of taming her. Why don't we take a page from Goofus and Gallant? Let's look at conversation.

-Goofus, when talking about such topics as politics and religion, always automatically agrees with the girl whenever she voices her opinion. If he says anything relevant to the subject at hand, it is nearly always in support of her theory. In essence, he echoes what she says and then lauds her for her brilliance and deep thinking while at the same time fawning over her.

-Gallant uses his brain and sees a discussion as an exciting opportunity to match mental wits with another human being. He talks about what he knows, and doesn't mouth off like an idiot when he doesn't understand something. If he disagrees, he tells the girl and they have an interesting discussion. It doesn't get heated, but he does ensure that it is a worthy conversation because there is a real back-and-forth going on. She deems him a worthy sparring partner as well as a man of ideas, and considered attractive to her. She likes the conversation and has a newfound respect for the man. She throws away Goofus' number when she gets home and starts sucking Gallant's dick. Goofus, meanwhile, jerks off with Icy Hot as his own personal punishment.

Get it? Girls don't want a P.R. representative. Women want a man who thinks for himself and ... well ... thinks before he speaks. You'd be surprised how rare this character trait is. Don't be afraid to disagree with her. It will assert your manhood and turn her on. Don't, however, get mean and too intense. You're trying to build a relationship and fuck her, not lead the debate team to the regionals! See it as playful fun and she will follow suit.

-When it is a holiday like Valentines or an Anniversary, Goofus brings home the obligatory Hallmark card, chocolates, dozen roses, and gifts, like clockwork. He kisses her lightly and they go to dinner at an upscale restaurant and share a bottle of wine. They go home and have some by-the-numbers missionary sex while Goofus leaves his socks on.

-Gallant surprises his sweetheart with presents

on random occasions, just because he was thinking of her. He gives her roses when he deems necessary but he also knows her favorite flowers and gets her those more often. When he gets her a card, he writes his own feelings inside instead of letting an international corporation with some dude in Paraguay voice his emotions. He makes the effort to keep special dates and occasions unique and fun, rather than falling in a rut. When he and his lover finally do go home, he fucks the shit out of her using the WT Technique and they both fall blissfully asleep.

Okay, you must get the point by now. It is not only perfectly fine to shower your woman with gifts -- it is a requisite. Don't worry about the fact that doing so is what a "clingy" or "desperate" guy might do. Women like a challenge but show her that you care about her. Don't, however, do it only when it is expected. Do you think a woman is going to soak her panties because you gave her a birthday present on her birthday and flowers for Valentine's Day? You have to be spontaneous, and throw her a bone when she least expects to receive something.

Spontaneity is important when it comes to relationships. Aside from random gift giving, try to be more spur of the moment when it comes to dates as well. Don't take her to Longhorn Steakhouse every Saturday, or you'll soon find that she's wrangled up a new buckaroo; one who takes her to Ruby Tuesday every Saturday! The same goes for the bedroom, and we'll get into that in just a second. For now, let's focus on being sweet, considerate and charming --- and I don't mean tasting good (F.Y.I., eat lots of fruits – especially pineapples and pineapple juice and your come will taste better than a Strawberry Tallcake from…choke…Ruby Tuesday).

Striking the right chord between adoring and arrogant isn't easy, but it is doable. What makes it work is the things we've been covering: Spontaneity, consideration, thoughtfulness and passion. Being sweet all the time will get you booted from her pussy faster than the Kentucky Derby winner. On the other hand, being consistently controlling and domineering will get old faster than a Carlos Mencia monologue. So shake it up and make sure that the majority of your behavior is that of a man who is in control. Remember, when it comes down to it, a woman will take a guy with initiative before a reflexive, malleable girly-man. Just don't beat the shit out of her, okay? Dennis Rodman got Carmen Electra by being a man but he lost her by whooping her ass. Get the picture?

Now let's getting into the nitty gritty sex stuff …

... IN THE BEDROOM

Fooling around in the bedroom is not only fun, but it is the best place to unleash untapped aggression and passion. Again, we'll want to look at the push and pull of tough love versus torrid physical passion. Let's use your dick as a symbolic "tool". We'll pretend your cock is a double edged sword. On one side is your troglodyte personality: your tough, domineering, manly man characteristics. On the other side of the sword is the sensitive, caring, loving aspect of you that whispers sweet nothings into her ear while you make gentle, nurturing love.

Would you only fuck a girl with half of your cock? Of course you wouldn't, unless she was a dwarf, and then nobody gives a shit how she feels. You'll need to slap her in the face with both sides of your dick. Think of tennis; hit her with a forehand and a backhand. The hand, in this case, is your dick. Women want both sides of a man –the soft side and the rough side, and there is only one-way to do it:

You're going to have to be good at the WT Technique if you want to truly tame a woman.

Girls may not be as shallow as us men, but they sure as shit want to come, damn it! You can be assertive, dominating, and respectful in all the right qualities in every aspect but if you can't fuck your gal right and satisfy her sexually, you're going to die miserable and alone. Hey,

I'm not trying to scare you … I'm trying to help you.

Many men never or only for a short period engage in foreplay ---they think sex is all about them. But rare is the woman who can come without foreplay. Give your tamee multiple orgasms so that she'll tell her friends about you and you can consequently get more ass. Foreplay is necessary for sheet-sliming orgasms.

You might be thinking that foreplay and eating pussy (a big part of foreplay) are the mark of a man who is submissive and is not in charge in the bedroom and otherwise. You would be wrong. Like we were discussing earlier, the bedroom is the perfect time for you to exercise your split personalities of the dominant caveman and the doting douche-bag. You can rock her world like the sexy stud you are while still nurturing her like Jude Law would do when he's not fucking a nanny.

The "fore" in "foreplay" indicates that it is an appetizer --- before the main course. Many people in fact see foreplay as the most important part of sex. Instead of divvying up parts of coitus into representations of dinner courses, think of the various aspects of sex as small "tapas" or plates like the ones eaten in Spain and other countries. Individual delicious meals that don't fill you up completely but, when taken together, form a wholly satisfying mastication adventure.

Don't, however, think of foreplay as a means to

make sex better for just the woman. Think of it as a necessary part of sex for both parties to get off. We men are like light bulbs. Turn us on and we go from cold to hot almost instantly. Women, on the other hand, are more like irons. Once you turn one on, you have to wait a while for it to heat up and then wait and wait after it is turned off for it to cool down again.

With foreplay, a happy medium is reached where men are slowed down, the woman is sped up, and we meet in the middle with fantastic ropes of man and lady come spraying willy-nilly in the air.

We're going to be delving into some pretty awesome stuff. With this guide, you'll be able to make your girl come so hard that her pubes get split ends. The caveat? You'll need to take some preliminary measures before taming her with your cock. Would you build a house without first laying out a foundation? Would you make a pizza without first making the dough?

This is a great time to remind her how beautiful you think she is. Sure, you're coming dangerously close to the threshold of Michael J. Fox's dad in Back to the Future, but there will be plenty of time to show dominance later. Consider yourself a snake in the grass, for now. In the meantime, why not show her how loving you are by giving her a massage. Make sure that you have some sensual oils handy. Oils help your fingers glide across her skin better while also making her feel better. Safflower is a good choice, as is coconut, because it is light and non-greasy.

Kissing may be kind of dull and lame, but women love it. You'll have to do quite a bit of this before the fun part, but remember that you'll be happier in the end when your woman is marveling over what a great fuck you were. You're probably thinking that kissing is more for douchey guys who are all soft and whatnot, but remember that you can control the kissing. Kiss her softly and gently of course but also feel free to kiss her forcefully. Grab her and kiss her like Stanley would kiss Stella (from the "Streetcar Named Desire" – It is implied in the play, that Stella is attracted to Stanley's passionate, animal nature, and that is why she stays with him). For those of you who are illiterate, kiss her like Sid would kiss Nancy ("Sid and Nancy" The movie is largely based on the mutually destructive, drug-and-sex filled relationship between Sid Vicious and Nancy Spungen).

While the two of you are getting your collective smooches on, start touching her body gently and as lightly as possible. This will give her more chills than a Cuban in Alaska. Pay attention to her breathing. When she changes from a normal pattern to more deep and relaxed breathing, she's getting ready to move on.

As you feel her breathing patterns begin to deepen, respond accordingly with more heavy touching focused more on her erogenous parts. Start kissing her gently around her nipples. Don't go right for the nipple, but instead kiss and lick gently around before you get there. Most girls love their breasts fondled and you can use your hands to keep her aroused up there as your mouth travels southward. Your face's destination is her pussy, but take the scenic route. Some girls love the thin skin on their inner thighs kissed and stroked. Plenty of girls are down for toe-sucking. You'll be able to tell the difference by her breathing or her vocalizations.

At this point, you're probably face to face with Mr. Vajayjay --- I didn't really say that … that's Oprah's line **(BTW, don't EVER let me catch you watching Oprah or Barbara Walters).**

As wonderful and magical as the woman's vagina is, however, there is an important little sucker above it called the clitoris or, as I call it, the head of her underground penis. To find this little bugger, pull apart those moist lips. You should see what looks like a little nipple. If it isn't aroused, it is small and looks almost like an ingrown hair. The more it is stimulated, though, the bigger it gets. This is the first Mecca of the female orgasm – this is where clitoral orgasms happen.

A clitoris is nothing but a tiny, tiny female cock head

From Britannica: In early embryonic life there are neither testicles nor ovaries but simply two undifferentiated organs called gonads that can develop either into testicles or ovaries. If the embryo has a Y-chromosome, the gonads become testicles; otherwise, they become ovaries. The testicles of the fetus produce androgens, and these cause the fetus to develop male anatomy. The absence of testicles results in the development of female anatomy. Animal experiments show that, if the testicles of a male fetus are removed, the individual will develop into what seems a female (although lacking ovaries). Consequently, it has been said that humans are basically female.

But this isn't a book about eating pussy – I'm sure you have done it many times and need no further instructions and can skip the next few pages. If you do need a quick guide about eating pussy … read on.

Clitoral stimulation is the only thing to focus on at this point. We'll get to the good stuff in a second, but for now let's stay on the clit. Below the clit is the urethra. That's the pee hole. You can stimulate this too, if you'd like. Many women like it, some don't. You'll also see the labia or "pussy lips". Feel free to kiss the pussy lips and rub them if you'd like, even if Pussy Lips sounds like the name of a bad Dick Tracy villain. Kiss around the general area until you get to the clit. Pull back the hood and start kissing it gently. I say gently because this is a very, very, very sensitive part of the woman's body. Use your tongue to play with it ever so slightly.

This is a great time to experiment. Don't lap it up like a Saint Bernard, though. Instead, think of your tongue as a hummingbird. If you're doing it right, you'll notice the clitoris swelling up in size. Remember not to keep doing the same motions repeatedly. You will want to switch it up. A good piece of advice is to trace the ABC's with your tongue on her clit. Don't say them out loud, of course, but keep it up and once you get to l m n o P!…she should be shivering in joy. Once she starts responding positively, now is the time to be repetitive. When you hit the motion that works for her, keep it up and she will start having an orgasm.

Don't forget to tell her how great she tastes. Even if it tastes like she fucked herself with a dead weasel, keep up appearances and act like you're munching on something divine. Girls are very self-conscious about their bodies and especially wary when it comes to their meat curtains. While you might care less about how she feels about her body, keep in mind that she will never be able to reach the orgasmic heights you're shooting for if she has the slightest qualms about her smells, tastes, and appearances.

This is also a great time to try out a little sixty-nine action. Many girls say that they're against 69'ing but usually it is just anti-pillow talk. No girl wants to go out and say that she likes sucking dick while getting her pussy eaten out, because that would be naughty and against the puritan values under which she was raised. The fact of the matter is that most girls like 69'ing precisely for the reason that it IS raunchy and dirty. If she doesn't like it, move on to other things.

Remember, also, that every girl is different. Some may like a gentle sucking motion, while others may deem it too intense. Improvise and listen to her, even though your ears will be muffled by a pair of thighs. Listen to her responses. You'll know if you're doing it right if she responds with joy. If you look up and see a Vanity Fair magazine in her hands, you're probably doing something wrong. One thing you'll definitely find out, though, is that too much forcefulness on the clit is a big no-no for almost any girl. How would you like a blowjob from a wolverine on acid? Biting, pulling, and any other kind of excessive force is out unless your girl is into genitorture – OK, I made that up.

NOW THE REAL FUN BEGINS...
THE WOMEN TAMED TECHNIQUE

You are about to learn a life changing sex technique. Sex will never be as it once was. Master the next few chapters and she will be tame as a kitten.

I am not a celebrity or a sex therapist. I am not a doctor so this book will not provide you with any form of medical jargon. You will not find a flow chart of the vagina or any type of medical advice that you could logically expect to find when you are speaking to a doctor. If you are looking for that kind of information, I am sorry, Google "woman's vagina" – you will get all the info you need. There is not a doctor in the world that will teach you, what you are about to learn.

I have never really kept track, but I have made love to (done, fucked, screwed ... whatever) over 50 women. I have no medical training but I can teach you plenty of things about a woman's body, her G-spot and the right way to stimulate it to create orgasm after mind blowing orgasm.

The average man believes a woman's body is like a whodunit mystery. When I started dating women, I was a dense dimwit. I thought the only thing I had to do was stick my dick in her pussy, jackhammer away as fast and hard as I could and we both would be happy.

First one smoking a cigarette wins.

Guess what? It does not work that way, not even close.

I have learned a great deal about the female anatomy. I have figured out what makes them explode with orgasmic pleasure. Most men have no clue how to master satisfying a woman. But you my friend, are about to learn the secrets of the G-spot and G-gasms.

What's a G-gasm?

Direct G-spot stimulation produces waves of G-spot orgasms or vaginal orgasms, AKA G-gasms. There are plenty of doctors that will swear there is no such thing as a "vaginal orgasm." These same experts will tell you that the only way to achieve female orgasm is by direct stimulation of the clitoris. Recent discoveries about the size of the clitoris - it extends inside the body – these nerve endings pass through the G-spot and connect to the spinal cord for transmission to the brain cells. As the G-spot is stimulated, it grows in size. Somewhat like a beneath the surface penis. How awesome is that?

Something like 75% of woman never or very rarely orgasm during intercourse – you are about to discover a way to make it happen every time.

How taming is that? Imagine YOU being able to make her come almost on demand. Think back, the last time you made love to your woman – did you satisfy her – did you really make her happy?

Did she orgasm during intercourse or did she fake it again? Visualize the power you have when you hold the keys to her orgasms.

What and where is the G-spot?

Back in 1950 there was a doctor Ernest Gräfenberg, M.D., who wrote the now famous article "The Role of Urethra in Female Orgasm."

Dr G was one smart dude. I like my analogy better of a beneath the surface penis. The clit is the only visible part of a women's underground penis with the rest of it being beneath the skin.

Thirty years later, Dr. Grafenberg's work was resurrected, the now famous spot he talked about in his article was christened the Grafenberg spot or G-spot for short.

The G-spot is located about 2-3 inches inside the vagina on the outside or anterior wall. That is it – no mystery, no nothing – that is the G-spot. It is not like the lost city of Atlantis or some beautiful, secret area run by the CIA. You can imagine your tamee's G-spot as almost opposite her clitoris but below the surface on the inside anterior wall of her vagina. When you have felt your way around in the vagina, you'll get to know the G-spot, as a "bump" surrounded by the smooth fleshy anterior wall. The "bump" will feel ribbed, almost like the roof of your mouth. Memorize the first sentence of this paragraph.

When you have some time, perform an Internet

search for the keyword – G-spot – look through the search results. You find articles from respected professors, so called authority magazines and publications about "The G-spot supposedly is a small, highly sensitive area on the anterior (front) wall of the vaginal cavity." Or you find questions from some poor guy asking about female ejaculation ...is it real? Is it dreaming? It's sad when some of these doctors are still standing around scratching their ass and wondering where the hell they went and hid that damn G-thang.

Can you imagine, a bunch of supposedly educated doctors sitting at a bar discussing the existence, or non-existence of the G-spot? All they have to do is find a willing partner, arouse her, stick a finger in her pussy – and there it is – about two to three inches in, on the anterior wall. Hmmm ....

An un-stimulated G-spot is only about the size of a pea and feels kind of like a dry roasted peanut shell. As the G-spot gets aroused and stimulated it swells to the size of a small walnut, giving you the clue that you not only found the spot but that it likes you! When the spot has swelled, the woman is in the big O zone and with more play; you will make her body sing.

In technical terms, the G-spot is a bundle of nerve clusters that trigger natural painkillers within a woman's body. These painkillers are the same endorphins that release during childbirth. The nerve endings are concentrated beneath the surface of the skin in a protective bundle, which allows for sensitivity and ability to handle fondling.

First as stressed earlier, get her sexually aroused. Don't ever stint on foreplay. Yeah, I know that you want to jump right in and get your fingers wet. Take your time; get her going first.

To locate the G-spot, face your tamee while she is lying on her back and insert your index or middle finger into her vagina. Then crook it upward toward yourself in a "come here" motion, sliding your fingertip along the top of the vagina until you find an area that is rougher than the rest of the vaginal wall. Make sure you have your fingernails clipped short before you do this - sharp fingernails will definitely spoil the moment. This rough or slightly ridged area is the G-spot, and touching it the first time, will often cause a woman to react with surprise and pleasure.

OK ... I found the G-spot ... Now what?

Now that we know where the G-spot is – it is time to have some fun. I have had great success with this method; the most important thing you can remember is that every woman is different. No woman has the same attitude towards this type of play. Take it easy – relax, have fun and make it fun for your partner. Communication is key; encourage her to talk.

Surprisingly, many sex manuals do not teach or

even talk about direct G-spot stimulation and G-spot orgasms. Everyone has heard about and knows about the G-spot; yet many researchers and so called experts, still refer to it as the "elusive" or "mythical" G-spot. Trust me, the G-spot is where I told you it is.

Despite both spots offering the ability to create mind blowing orgasms the G-Spot is very different from the clit. In the beginning, you might treat the two in a similar fashion with some soft touching and light rubbing. However, when you have stimulated the G-Spot enough to get it going, that is when the real fun begins. A good guideline to remember will be to show the clit some mercy but to be merciless when it comes to the G-Spot! Within reason, most women will appreciate a harsher approach to the G-Spot.

I'll remind you again … the most important thing to remember is that every woman is different. If you move into dating and sexual types of relationships assuming that all women are the same, you are
going to be mistaken. No woman has the same attitude and anatomy. While their anatomy may indeed be similar, they are not all the same, not by a long shot, and good communication is the cornerstone of great sex.

Prepare your hands for this erotic experience. Scrub your hands well. Long manicured fingernails may look good, but not for what you are about to do. Keep the nails short and filed smooth. Before you begin the activities, to help prevent rough, dry hands in any weather, be sure to routinely massage your favorite hand cream thoroughly into your hands. The massaging action stimulates blood circulation throughout the hands and promotes the absorption of conditioners into your skin. Apply your cream often, especially after washing your hands or after submerging them in water. Your tamee will really appreciate your prep work.

There are only two actual "rules" for the WT Technique.

Rule number one is to have the lady use the bathroom before you begin. Stimulation to the G-spot will give her the sensation that she needs to urinate. However, if she knows she just did, it is less likely to bother her. The urination sensation does not last for a long time, though you don't want to end up having a stream of her urine land on you. You water sports guys might not mind this, it would be a deal breaker for most!

Rule number two is probably more important than rule number one. As we talked before, start with foreplay – kissing, touching, hot oil rub – whatever the two of you are in the mood for. Do everything you normally would do to turn her on, do not go directly to the WT Technique. This is essential; you must get her going first. This is especially important the first few times you attempt G-gasms. Lots of oral, dip your cock in her for a bit, try different positions, more oral and fingers and only then when she is about to burst, try G-spot manipulation. She should be fully stimulated and the whole vagina area engorged with her at the point of begging for more.

Some guys like to give their ladies an oral clitoral orgasm first, I recommend that you bring her close to orgasm, but don't let her cum. Use your talents and toys to bring her to the edge of orgasm over and over again. Many women are the one-orgasm types; their bodies are trained and are satisfied after one orgasm. Skip the clitoral orgasm; make her desperate for release. If she is moaning, dripping wet, and almost incoherent she wants to cum so much, now is the time to go G-spot thwacking full-time.

The Women Tamed ™ Technique

Have her lay on her stomach with her rear up in the air and her face leaning against some pillows. Make sure to have her legs at a comfortable width apart. Put a couple of pillows under her hips to get her tush up in the air. Position yourself at her side or between her legs.

Insert your thumb, thumbprint side down, in her pussy. Press the thumb downwards so that you are pressing towards the pillows under her hips. You will find the G-Spot right about where your thumbprint is. I know it sounds simple, because it is! There really is nothing to finding the G-spot. Keep in mind everybody's body is different.

If she looks, or says she is uncomfortable, back off for a while, go back to doing "comfortable" things. You can always try again later or the next session. The first time is the hardest – after that, it is easy to find and play with the G-spot – insert thumb, press down (this is with the lady on her stomach, butt up). Feel around for a smallish, rough bump that is bigger than a pea. The size will depend on the woman and the amount of foreplay. As she becomes more and more excited and the G- spot is stimulated, it will grow in size to about the size of a walnut. The G-spot is going to feel rougher than the smooth texture of the inner vagina walls.

Now that you found the spot, start rubbing. Start to rub in a back and forth or side to side motion. At this point, the key thing to remember is not to rub it too hard. You will be able to feel the spot thicken and grow against your thumb. Once this happens you will be able to increase your movement and get rougher with it. Rub it, as if you are trying to get a stain off your jeans.

Any guy that treats the clit rough will usually get a kick in the balls. After a clit stimulated orgasm, be it manually or with the tongue, even look at her clit and a woman will push you away. The G-spot is different. Once triggered and excited, do not treat it as a clit. In the excited state, the G-spot likes abuse – treat it rough.

Beat an engorged, fully eager penis with a hammer and a man would say, " Wow – that feels great." The G-spot is similar. Be gentle with the clit – be rough with the G-spot.

As the G-Spot continues to swell, she will get the feeling that she has to urinate. However, that was the reason for having her take a pee before hand. I always ignore the request – a good smack on the ass works well here. The "have to pee" feeling will go away in a little while.

When the G-Spot gets excited and swells, it puts pressure on the bladder giving the woman a sensation of needing to tinkle. This feeling only lasts for about 30 seconds, and then subsides. Many newbie tamees become uncomfortable at this point; I assure you the feeling will change to a highly sexual pleasurable feeling.

While many women don't have to be asked to talk, and are more than willing to tell you how to rub their G-spot, I have been with just as many who need that little extra push to talk. To find out if you are in the right spot, just ask. You may find she wants you to move to the left or right. She might want you to be rougher and faster or slower and softer. Try rubbing side to side, up and down, "punch" it, rub round and round, tap the spot like a tiny drum, poke at it like you are trying to push it, jab at it like you are trying to pick it up with a fork, press on it with no movement, bring out the dentist's drill, vacuum cleaner, or chainsaw ... whatever it takes.

After a few minutes you should hear the mind-blowing madness which will be your woman having a G-gasm. The first time I watched this I could not believe my eyes. My life changed with one G-Gasm! She'll be bucking and pushing against your hand with all she has, moaning and screaming, she'll cum so hard she may squirt all over your hand.

Not everyone will have quick, fast and successful results – some couples will have staggering G-gasms within minutes – other couples try everything short of sacrificing a goat - we are not the same. The couples having trouble need to be persistent and they need to persevere and eventually, after many attempts, they will be like "WOW – WHAT THE FUCK – THAT WAS AMAZING." Once the first G-gasm is unleashed, all hell breaks loose. Whatever the immediate results are, remember that getting there is 90% of the fun.

A word of warning: Never try this method with your tamee sitting on your face. If you do not drown from the pussy juice, you will certainly have a broken nose.

The Next Level of the WT Technique

After the first G-gasm, you can trigger additional G-Gasms within seconds to a minute. After she cums the first time, start rubbing again, just as hard as before. The G-gasms will happen repeatedly. Of course, each woman has a different tolerance for this, so you will want to watch it carefully. Some women cannot take the rigorous abuse of her body so often. If she

89

cannot stand many G-gasms, don't worry, because as sessions continue, the need and ability to achieve multiple G-gasms seems to progress. You will have her experiencing 10, 20 or more G-gasms per session in no time! Again, do not be gentle – unless of course she asks.

When you have her at that point – DO NOT STOP. The whole idea of using this technique is that you can keep going. Wait until you see her reaction when you make her G-gasm for the first time.

Now that she knows the feeling of a G-gasm, it will be easier and easier to make her G-gasm repeatedly. The way to really blow her mind is make her G-gasm like that for 30 or 60 seconds straight, and then give her a rest to catch her breath and then start again ... and again ... and then some more.

It is like finding the key to the vault. Her body will know what it feels like from then on. Marathon sessions will be fun, but "quickies" in mall parking lots, or before the kids wake up for breakfast are a scream too. Once the vault has been opened, reaction time can be almost instantaneous if she is horny and you have 30 seconds to get your thumb in there and give her a good rub.

This is much better than just FUN. Most women do not have any idea that they are capable of such sexual energy and multiple orgasms. After five or six G-gasms, they start to look at you with amazement. Like, "How the hell are you doing that to me?" I do not give them any mercy – nor should you. "Torture" them with G-gasm after G-gasm. You my friend, hold the keys.

FEMALE EJACULATION/SQUIRTING

Like mirages, rainbows, shooting stars and other nature masterpieces, female ejaculation has provided amazement and controversy. Many woman and researchers believe that because the fluids expelled during female ejaculation come from the urethra, that really the woman is experiencing loss of bladder control. In other words – she peed a little.

Men take ejaculation for granted. It is the "runny-prize" of sex – and the source of your future heritage. The only conceivable purpose of female ejaculation is for pleasure – very intense pleasure at that. This method can produce ejaculation when performed on a willing partner.

In some porno movies, there is a scene where the woman is shown ejaculating a clear or milky fluid. Is it real pussy cum? Is it trick editing? Is it pee? That is a lot of questions ... I think it is real.

I did a lot of research on female ejaculation, or squirting. I studied videos of women cumming, and I have read scientific articles. Hell, I am man enough to admit it - I even picked up a copy of Cosmopolitan Magazine a time or two just to try to figure out how to please a woman (don't let me catch you reading Cosmo).

The tissue surrounding the female urethra fills

with blood during sexual arousal, as the penis does in men. This results in the tissue becoming firm to the touch. Researchers believe that female cum is produced by the Skene's glands. Skene's glands are located in the urethra. These glands are similar in makeup to a man's prostate gland. Female cum is made of prostatic acid phosphatase, the same chemical secreted by the prostate gland and found in semen, minus the sperm of course. Do you remember my "underground penis" analogy? This indicates that a woman's ejaculation is similar in composition to semen.

Woman who experience G-gasms also enter the wonderful world of "squirting." Not all women, all the time experience ejaculation, some experience it sometimes, some women never squirt. Most females have the ability to ejaculate, but often do not and usually squirting is a taboo subject and not discussed openly. When was the last time you heard of anyone discuss "depositing her load" over a few beers?

In the past, medical doctors told ladies seeking advice about bodily fluids that they are incontinent, rather than told they are ejaculating. That led to shame and humiliation. What girl would want to be known as a bed wetter? Instead of enjoying the ejaculation sensation, many women believed they had "golden-showered" their partner. Many men thought they had been "golden throated" while giving oral to their lady friend. Many females will admit to having had an experience where they believed they had "leaked" during sex. The feeling of ejaculating is similar to peeing, a shower of warm wet liquid and a feeling of release.

Be prepared for the flow of ejaculate. If you are into "water sports," this is going to be a huge turn on for you. Do not react like "what the fuck is that – did you piss yourself???" because that will make it embarrassing for both of you. It is a normal body function. Make the tamee feel comfortable, or she will dry up like a mud puddle and so will your sex life. You laugh, but I swear, if she thinks she peed herself during sex, she will lose her sexual high completely.

You will be amazed at the amount of fluid her body can produce. Up to two cups of expelled ejaculate can slather your sheets during a love making session. The amount varies, as does the force of ejection. Sometimes, the your hand will get soaking wet, and other times her spunk will bathe the soles of your feet. How awesome is that? This is a new slant on the question of "who sleeps on the wet spot?"

A Few WT Technique Guidelines

Most women can ejaculate but many do not. In the same way that all women can orgasm even though some do not ever achieve climax, be it through bodily or psychological blockage, or in-experience. Playing with her G-spot for hours at a time does NOT necessarily mean she is going to ejaculate. That happens with some ladies some times.

Don't get bummed if it doesn't happen – she is still having G-gasms and having a good time. She doesn't need to squirt. Again, some women will squirt a little; some will gush a lot; some will not spray at all; and some will shoot sometimes.

Back when you were a young teenager and started to spank your monkey, it didn't take you long to produce a load of jizz. The climax in woman is much more complex, but once they start they do not stop. Unlike men, there is more to follow. Give her a few minutes and she will be filling up like a Hummer's gas tank. Each subsequent G-gasm will deliver a different volume of liquid in all directions and velocities. This can range from a trickle of one ounce to an almost a chaotic cupful. Don't worry about the juices drying up, there is always plenty more.

As a rule, guys do not care who they cum with. For the ladies, it starts with the partners being compatible. Ladies that do ejaculate are conscious of "showering their lover." Men could care less, and prefer to "shower" in a flamboyant manner, i.e. facials, in her mouth, on her tits, you know, we like to make it dramatic – "WHOA BABY –check it out, that shot went five feet and landed on the alarm clock!"

Ejaculate fluid is different from the normal "pussy juice" or "love juices." Love juices are a natural lube for the vagina that appears with arousal. Squirting or female ejaculation comes from the urethra or pee hole. Since female cum originates and emanates from the urethra, the fluid is mixed with a little pee.

Men cannot pee and cum at the same time. When a man is about to ejaculate, the opening to the bladder closes, making peeing impossible. A woman on the other hand, (so to speak) is able to ejaculate and pee at the same time. Frequently that feeling of peeing and oncoming orgasm are confused. That is why I stressed earlier that your tamee should use the little ladies room, before you start your sexual activity. You do not want your lady to think about peeing – you want her thinking about G-gasms and ejaculations.

Getting your lady friend to squirt for the very first time is like obtaining a PhD in sexology. The building of the ejaculation feels like the desire to pee. As soon as the urethra starts to tingle, second nature kicks in and she contracts her PC muscles to stop the flow of urine. She must oppose the contraction and try to squeeze out, as if trying to pee. This is not an easy concept, in that contraction of the PC muscles will actually stop the ejaculation from building. As squeezing the base of the cock and thinking momentarily of Mickey Mantle's batting average postpones cumming in men, "squeezing in" postpones female ejaculation. "Squeezing out" instead of "squeezing in" is a major barrier for many ladies trying to ejaculate. Practice will overcome the barrier.

OK guys, you have been warned, don't forget to use the biggest towels you can find; you don't want your mattress to start smelling weird after a while.

Working the WT Technique

Peeing - the subject of most emails. Make sure she goes for a good pee before you start your activities, so she knows her bladder is empty. She will get that "I have to pee" feeling as the G-spot swells with excitement. That "I have to pee" sensation precedes huge multiple G-gasms and puddles of cum. Help her relax and accept the new sensations, mix it up with a little oral, while you are "training" the G-spot. Often the first G-gasm will happen when she least expects it. After that, it is easy to "rinse and repeat."

After the first G-gasm, give her a short 10 – 30 second break, this gives her time to catch her breath but not long enough for her to come down from her sexual high. Then proceed with more rubbing – the same way you did for the first orgasm. Keep doing what you were doing – don't piss her off – she'll poke a hot stick in your eye when you are sleeping. If she is seriously overwhelmed and does not want anymore, this gives her the time to let you know.

You are in control of her orgasms; you can allow them to come full on, or hold them back. Once you make her cum once or twice, you can continue this cycle until she begs you to stop, or until she goes into an orgasmic coma of sorts.

♥ If the tamee has an active job, you might want to save this activity for special events and weekends. I can guarantee that she will be sore and have a somewhat hard time walking when the next day rolls around.

♥ If there is not an immediate response from the lady, take it slowly; work her with foreplay so that she is as horny as you can make her. Work her orally and maybe even with little intercourse, and then try the WT Technique again. If she doesn't respond, go back to something else; get her near orgasm, then back to the Technique. You are in no rush – have fun.

♥ When rubbing, vary the pressure. Of course don't hurt your tamee, but it takes a firm hand and fingers, and a surprising amount of pressure to produce a G-gasm.

♥ This will become addictive to her. It will make your tamee feel subservient to your sexual prowess.

♥ Many women have expressed to me that a G-gasm is a mind-blowing experience. Their entire body receives a sense of relief. If your tamee has never experienced this, you may want to give her more than a minute between each G-Gasm. Wait until she seems to have caught her breath. Once she can breathe normally again, it is time for round two, three, four, or ten.

♥ Do not worry about the size of your fingers because like the size of your penis it is going to have little to do with the amount of pleasure she ends up receiving. Length has nothing to do with this. Instead, you will be concentrating on the amount of pressure you are using and not how much you are shoving inside her.

♥ Experiment with just slightly different positions of your finger(s). The G-spot is easy to miss, and if you are off just a bit the rubbing will still feel good for the lady, but won't produce G-gasms.

♥ Try edging, to increase the intensity just a little bit more; learn the flow of her G-gasms and stop before she has one. Start rubbing her and get her close to G-gasm, then stop. Give her a minute for a breather and then go back to rubbing. Leave your fingers/thumb inside her but do not move them. When you finally rub her off, she will be bucking her hips and grinding back on you like a stripper whore!

♥ If you have never experienced female ejaculation, it may appear that she is squirting something. Don't worry! It is not pee or anything. It is a good thing, especially for the tamee! Some women become embarrassed after ejaculating the first time – they think they peed in bed – but it is not pee. With G-gasms, some ladies will ejaculate – go with the flow, so to speak. Bring a towel … or a bucket. Guys remember, keep rubbing past the "I got to pee" feeling, she is ready to G-gasm!

♥ Water based lubes sometimes help.

♥ Once the tamee has experienced a few G-gasm sessions, her body seems to know what to expect and doesn't need as much foreplay to trigger a series of G-gasms. You can warm her up a little, insert thumb/finger rub and give her three or 4 massive G-gasms. It is a great way for a little quickie before she heads off to work.

♥ Most   tamees are capable of G-gasms. Barring surgery and birth defects, all women have the correct "plumbing" in place to make G-gasms happen. This doesn't mean that the WT Technique will work on all women 100% of the time. A combination of factors prevents G-gasms from happening. Fear, being the biggest culprit. Fear of "being dirty," fear of letting loose, fear of urinating and fear of losing control – these fears can be overcome. But birth defects, a cesarean section, hysterectomy or other surgeries may make it impossible to achieve G-gasms.

♥ Sex is not about the destination but rather the journey. If she's enjoying it, keep it up. With time, you will make progress. I receive countless emails from couples saying, "doesn't work …," "we can't …," "it seems that …," or "didn't work." Later, all of a sudden I receive, "WOW … unbelievable." Don't get frustrated and give up … keep at it, you will not be disappointed.

Losing Control

Keep an eye on your tamee, especially the first few times you try the Technique. If your lover is used to being in control, then the total loss of control that comes with G-gasms may make her uneasy. She will still be able to enjoy herself, but women do lose control during these sessions. Some women get scared – scared at the intensity, frequency and total loss of control of the orgasms. Many tamees will ask you to stop until they become comfortable with the Technique.

This is where you have to decide whether it is time to hold her down and proceed or to go on to other activities.

Often when she is at the "scared" point, her G-gasm is seconds away. If you can force a few more rubs, she will have no choice but to cum, and then you can repeat the process.

Always be loving, understanding and supportive to your tamee, but don't let her call all the shots. Sometimes, even if you are usually a pussy-whipped boy toy, this is a great time to slap her ass, pull her hair, tell her she's a slut and a whore and tell her to shut the fuck up and that you are in charge now.

Pull this off and she will know the meaning of respect.

You Are So Naughty

Add in a little BDSM activities during your G-Spot marathons. This will really heat things up. A few well-placed spankings with your hand or a paddle will do. In addition to this, tie her down and control how many G-gasms she has! What a nice little mixture – the kinkiness of a G-spot rubbing together with a little bit of submissiveness – awesome. Be careful, this might be too intense for some tamees.

Edging

Edging is the art of bringing yourself or your tamee to the point of orgasm, but being able to hold yourself back. It takes some practice and you need strong PC muscles. As outlined in the "female ejaculation" section, Kegel exercises strengthen your PC muscles.

A typical regimen for a strong and healthy PC muscle; clasp and hold tight for ten seconds – gradually increase the time interval and the length of sets. Practice Kegels persistently – short sets in the beginning, then gradually, over months, increasing both the number of Kegels you do a day and the amount of time you are able to hold a series of very long Kegels.

When edging, build yourself up to the point of orgasm, then stop or switch to something less stimulating. Practice this while masturbating. The advantage of building up and stopping is that it pumps your entire system. When you finally do have an orgasm with this method, you will see what I mean. It is the most powerful thing you can do.

Most women usually take longer and need more stimulation than men. Bring your tamee almost to the point of orgasm five or six times, she will begin to shake and quiver, and will beg you to let her cum. When she finally does cum, she will cum like the dirty little slut that she is.

I love teasing and playing by bringing the tamee right up to the edge of a G-gasm, and then stop rubbing for a few moments. After a few times of having her on edge, I will let her have a G-Gasm. After the first one, you can expect a flood. Prolonging the first G-gasm seems to make the following ones almost intolerably intense and recur quickly.

NOW FUCK HER

The best part about this technique is that after the first G-gasm, the carry-over effect is real and may last for hours. Most women can achieve another G-gasm with only a few well-placed rubs. Wait 10 seconds to 30 seconds, rub a little more and it would all happen again ... and again ... and again. That is what makes this Technique so awesome and powerful.

Most woman experience clitoral orgasms, either by direct manual stimulation or oral stimulation. A G-gasm is like an orgasm on the inside. Once you awaken the G-spot with your finger(s), give her G-spot some cock action.

Try this ...

After a few manual – meaning finger – G-gasms, position yourself between her knees, while she is on her back. Spread her knees apart and hold her still. Make sure she is wet, or lubed up, and insert the head of you cock in her pussy. Instead of thrusting like a Chippendale dancer, rock back and forth gently, aiming your cock to stroke the top of her pussy. An upward curve to your dick, so it rubs right up along the top, or front of the vagina, makes the sensation for her even better. You might want to push her knees up and back towards her to get a better angle.

After a few minutes of this, she will slip into another world – maybe another universe. After her first cock induced G-gasm, she might appear to go limp - just keep going of course! Within perhaps 30 seconds, she will go into some scene from Psycho; she will buck uncontrollably. Hold onto her legs, you don't want her getting away, because you want to do it again, and again … and then once more.

After you do this to a woman, your confidence level soars to a new high. Your lovemaking ability seems to get better and better. Using this Technique, with practice, you will be able to give her G-gasms almost on command.

Penis size doesn't matter; remember the G-spot is only two or three inches inside the vagina. You can have a three-inch dick and still massage her G-spot.

After you "awaken" and warm up the G-spot manually with a G-gasm or two, stimulation via penetration produces waves of G-gasms. After the show is finally over, she will relent and be yours. Think of it like breaking a horse. It fights all it can but eventually a talented rider will become the master of the beast.

Doggy style works well too …

Remember that you don't necessarily have to be on top to make this work. You may wish to let her hop on top and find the right spot on her own. If, however, you'd like to keep dominion over domination, nothing spells "I'm your master" better than doggy style. Not only is doggy style the best position for G-spot stimulation, but it also is the number one position for showing dominance.

Many women in fact don't like being fucked doggy style because it is so inherently demeaning. These women usually are more bark than bite when it comes to being fucked like a dog (pardon the pun), and actually would just love a man to bend them over and fuck them like a dirty, disgusting animal. You might wish to put some pillows under her hips so that her ass is at the perfect angle for G-spot stimulation. Experiment around a little bit until you're at just the right position. Try to get your pelvis up higher than her ass and then thrust downward or along her front pussy wall. The tamee will let you know when you're at just the right angle.

Taming a woman requires work in all areas but taming a woman in the bedroom is by far the most fun, wouldn't you say? Making her orgasm through G-spot stimulation is great because you are the one in control. Whether she likes it or not (and she does, of course), she has to submit to you. You are the pleasure giver and you can take it away just as easily. What is even better is that she can't even control herself at this point! Her screams and shivers and spasms are beyond her range. You have officially dominated this woman and have left her a sopping pile of flesh that can be molded in whatever way you wish, but don't stop now! We've only just begun! Experiment a little! This is where the fun begins … Slap her ass, yank on her hair, call her a slut, and tell her that you are the one in charge. If she asks you to stop, don't do it. Keep at it and she'll thank you later. Try out different angles and techniques, now that you know where the G-spot is and what to do with it.

If you fuck your girl just right, she will look at you in a whole new light. Instead of just another schmuck, you'll be, in her eyes, some kind of prodigy; a symphony conductor who can elicit screams of the highest pitch in her. While there are some tried and true tips that will help you to become superman a lot of the work will have to be done by you, because all girls are different and different things get them off.

Anal Play

I've found that the best time to bring up anal is when the tamee is a bit drunk and horny. Naturally, you'll want to start with some good old fashioned G-spot play and fucking before dipping a finger or two into the abyss. Make sure she is warmed up.

The butt-hole is not just an exit hole. It can be the source of a heck of a lot of pleasure for a woman, as well as being a great way for you to show dominance. First, let me stress this point: If she doesn't want you going in there, stay the fuck outta there. If, however, she is not completely against the idea, try sliding a finger in there while you're fucking her. The asshole is full of nerve endings that love to be stimulated. Having a dick in the pussy and a finger or two up the shitter gives women the feeling of being "filled" and it can really get them off in wondrous ways.

You don't necessarily have to be UP there, either, for the pleasure receptors to kick into gear. Many girls like to have their button rubbed and played with, without having anything inserted up there. Know what else they like? Having it licked! Yes, go ahead and get those gasps out. Licking ass is VERY kinky and, lest you think it is something a submissive pussy boy might do, analingus will actually assert your domination even more so, because you can bet that you likely won't be ASKED to do it; not the first time at least.

Make sure you have lube handy. Repeat: Lube. Not lotion, spit, or love juices. Astroglide or Vaseline is just fine. Remember to use a rubber, also. Go slow. A good piece of advice is to let her get on top. This will allow her to control the pace of insertion so that neither of you will be in too much pain. If you really want to assert your dominance over her, don't use a condom and don't come inside of her. Instead, pull out and make her go ass-to-mouth - also know as going from the shitter-to-the-spitter. Most girls think this is the nadir (or is it apex?) of disgustingness but, like we've discussed, some women like to be demeaned by a man.

Autogasms

Many women and men have written in to talk about something amazing called an autogasm. The autogasm is a new phenomenon that occurs when the body is in a blissful state from receiving so much pleasure. Mini G-gasms continue for hours after any sexual activity has ended. A woman that is able to have them will never forget them.

I have never been with a woman that has experienced autogasms, but from talking to couples that have had the pleasure, they are a series of mini G-gasms that recur as the lady is coming down from her sexual high. In all cases, the love making sessions were long and intense, lasting more than two hours with the lady experiencing 20 or more G-gasms in that period.

Again, not all couples encounter autogasms. Imagine your lady going to work after a 20 something G-gasm session.

"Roche, why are you walking so funny?" asked Mr. Klumpkin, her boss at work.

"Oh, I don't know … hubby and I were … oh my gosh … what the fuuuu … oh man … no way … this is not … oh goooowwddd …."

"Roche, what's the matter? Can I get you some water?"

"Towel … please."

CURING ALL YOU MINUTEMEN

As we've been discussing, the bedroom is the prime spot to fully realize your dominant self and the best place to tame your woman. This is where you can bring shock and awe to your woman and make her yours in every facet. Giving your woman the best sex of her life will automatically make her tame as a pet dog because you will become the bringer of joy and dominance. Now you know what it takes to bestow upon your tamee multiple moments of rapture inducing orgasmic glee, but you lack the necessary duration it requires.

In other words … what if you come too fast to get her off?

This is the bane of many a man and can spell certain doom in your quest for taming the fairer species. Do you honestly think your woman will allow you dominion over her heart and soul if you blow your load within thirty seconds of unclasping her bra? Coming too soon just gives her more time to laugh, get dressed, and go to her friends house to tell her about how you come too soon and what a lousy lay you are!

I can't let that happen to you … here's what you MUST do …

There are several ways for you to stave off an unwanted climax. The most popular and overused way is to think about baseball. This is hackneyed sitcom fodder but it might work for some of you. The problem, though, is that while you're imagining baseball, you're subconsciously realizing that you're thinking about baseball because you've got this hot, naked bitch under you. All of a sudden, the image of A-Rod will do nothing to keep a lid on your syringe (no offense there A-Rod). You'll think about baseball and then you'll think about ballpark dogs. Next you'll think about buns and you'll be right there in the same pickle.

Imagining something else CAN work in some instances, though. Try thinking about your grandmother when you feel like you're about to come. If that doesn't work, think about your grandmother sucking your grandfather's dick. If that doesn't work, think about your mom eating out your grandmother. Just keep thinking about family members and you should be able to stave off the inevitable for a little longer.

Another great trick is to think about the real world. If you have a pressing deadline at work, for instance, just thinking about it for a few seconds can allow you to worry just enough to take your mind off the action and keep thrusting for a bit longer. If you owe somebody money and they're particularly angry about it, imagine the beating you'll receive in the near future. You get the idea.

Another great tip involves your...well...tip. Pulling out and pinching your dickhead with a thumb on the top and a finger on the bottom can help keep you from coming. Do this discreetly, when changing positions or something similar. Squeezing your balls fairly hard works too, but it isn't for everyone. Flicking the balls is a similar trick that works well for some people, and not as well for others.

I know it's a little bit of a sissy-man position, but being on the bottom works in staving off an on-coming orgasm. If you're on top and you feel like you're about to blow your load, try flipping over and putting her on top.

Ever hear of Kegels?

Kegels exercises are working out the muscles that you contract when you hold your piss in because you don't want to stop at that gas station where those cretins are hanging out. They are also the same muscles that keep you from coming. Try it now. Act like you want to stop your piss. Feel that contraction? Those are your PC muscles, which stand for pubococcygeus. To master when and where you shoot your scrotal soda your PC muscles need a workout.

So how do you strengthen these muscles?

It's easy and far more entertaining than doing crunches. Do these exercises **every day for the rest of your life**. Within a couple of weeks, you'll notice a marked difference in your ability to contain your penis Pepsi from shooting out at inopportune moments.

You can do these exercises anywhere: while driving; waiting in line at the bank; waiting in line at the grocery store; do them while at work, etc. Once you are skilled at Kegel exercises, you should be able to do them without anyone else knowing what you are doing.

Go to your local adult shop and pick up a few cock rings. They don't have to be the expensive type (no metal) – a couple of bucks at most. The "o-rings" at Home Depot work well also. Buy a few different sizes so that you can get the right inside diameter. Cock rings engorge your penis by stopping the blood flow out of your cock. Cock rings also help prevent premature ejaculation. As an added bonus, cock rings give your dick a nice fat, chubby look. They don't make your cock any longer, but a properly fit cock ring will make your meat "girthier."

A Kegel exercise program along with wearing a cock ring is the most powerful method for ending embarrassing premature ejaculation. You'll literally be able to "turn off the hose" – very POWERFUL.

PC Muscles – Kegels For Men

Here's a simple set of exercises that can bring back a firmer erection, create mind-blowing orgasms and give you the ability to "turn off the hose". Strong PC muscles give you the ability to stop the flow of ejaculate during orgasm, thereby delaying and prolonging your fun. When you finally do ejaculate, you might splatter the headboard behind you.

To find your PC muscle, start to urinate then stop in midstream. If you have trouble stopping the flow of urine, you probably also have weak orgasms and premature ejaculation.

Do not exercise while urinating.

PC clamps: squeeze and release, start by holding for five seconds and then gradually increase the time. Start with "sets" of ten, and build up to sets of 100 or more. Do these every day for the rest of your life. This is a great exercise while you are driving or standing on line at the grocery store.

Long squeeze: Hold your PC muscle compressed tight for a count of twenty. Build up the strength to 30 or 50 count.

Slow squeeze: Tighten the PC muscle as slowly as you possibly can – repeat as often as you can.

You can do these exercises anywhere and at any time, there is absolutely no excuse to neglect your exercises. No one will know that you are squeezing, unless of course you keep smiling like a dumb ass while doing them, thinking about the next WT session.

PC Muscles – Kegels for Tamees

Kegel exercises were originally created to help women strengthen their PC muscles to help stop urinary incontinence after childbirth, when the PC muscle has been stretched out. The Kegel exercise turns out, has sexual benefits also.

There are three reasons she should do her Kegel exercises.

First, a strong PC muscle will help her overcome the "have to pee" feeling during the WT Technique.

Second, when the PC muscle is stretched out, less of the vagina and G-spot area is in direct contact with the penis and therefore receives less stimulation – less fun for her and you.

Thirdly, a well-toned PC muscle will give her a powerful ejaculation. Keep the PC muscle exercised with Kegels – she will have greater blood flow to the area, and the greater ability to become aroused and feel sexual pleasure.

The great thing about doing Kegel exercises is that no one knows you are doing them. While you can do all sorts of variations, the basic female Kegel exercises are:

Contract your PC muscles. Hold initially for a count of five; build up gradually to a count of twenty. Repeat ten times and practice daily. Like with all muscles you are better off building the

PC muscle slowly and regularly.

Let the Taming Begin ...

Remember: Act like yourself, bring out your personality or you are destined to fail. It is inevitable. That doesn't, however, mean that you can't change your overall being in order to be better able to have control over a woman. If you've consistently failed with women in the past, it has likely been because you have been too "into" her. Comedians aren't joking when they say that women are full of shit, insane and they only love romantic guys in romantic comedies. You can get away with that shit if you're Dylan Mcdermott or Dermot Mulroney (Dylan's mutated twin).

Women love three things in a man: Confidence, a challenge, and great sex. Bowing to their every whim will be your ruin. You have to assert control if you want to keep her, even if it goes against your every instinct.

You may not like the way romance works, but you can't change it. What, are you going to take it up with Darwin? We've advanced very little as a species. The past few thousand years of human evolution has been a queef in the grand span of the universe. You'll have to find your inner Neanderthal and embrace him. Back in those days, dominance was everything. Without it, we wouldn't have evolved as a species. It wasn't until the colonization of Bedrock that men started to lose their traits of domination and

allow their wives to lock them out of the house and throw their men around by their thumbs.
You have to face the facts - your failure with women stems from your shrugging off the nature of evolution.

Many woman find this Training Method scary or uncomfortable. They have been used to controlling everything --- including YOU, and now they cannot – you are in charge.

Refer to the sex part in this book as often as you need to. Sex is a drastically important factor when it comes to staking your claim as the Alpha Male.

Also, try to monitor HOW forceful you are being, in the bedroom and otherwise. You can't be too aggressive or you'll scare her off. When you're questioning your level of dominance, refer to the section on sensitivity and how to express your softer side.

Now go get out there, drag her by her hair back to the cave, and make me proud!

On to part two …

Bonnie's Gang Publishing is proud to present:

Element-X !

How to Meet, Date and Sleep With Killer Chicks

ELEMENT-X

Published by Bonnie's Gang Publishing, New York

http://BonniesGang.com/

FOR THE MILLIONS OF MEN THAT DON'T GET LAID ENOUGH.

Forward

Today I'm able to meet women no matter where I go. My fear of approaching is gone and I'm comfortable in virtually any group setting and soon, so will you.

In fact, I enjoy engaging women and challenging them *in a good way*. I like making women laugh. If you had told me ten years ago that I would have ended up on hundreds of dates with a variety of women I would have laughed you out of the room.

A mistake that I made as a young pick up artist was that I focused too much on technique in my early days. There's nothing wrong with focusing on technique, in fact, I encourage it because it gives men somewhere to start.

My problem was that I focused 99% of my efforts on technique and 1% of mindset. If you were to ask me today what's far more important than technique I would answer that **ELEMENT-X** destroys technique any day of the week**.**

Element-X is far more than mere confidence. It's also far more than simple mastery of technique(s).

Once a man has Element-X he no longer relies on technique. He simply relies on **who he is at any given moment.** It's that thing that women refer to when they say *"there's* *something about him that I can't describe..."*

In the next section, I explain exactly what Element-X is. I just want you to know that **YOU can attain it** because it is a **learned behavior**.

I'm going to give you all the necessary ingredients to make it work. I'm going to give you the blueprint, but you have to follow it, I can't do that for you. So, get ready to discover what 99% of all men don't know.

Then I want you to think about the 1% that do might know this but the majority of them don't apply it with any consistency. If you can master these principles, you will have very little competition out there and the ladies will love you for it.

Let's do it...

Please visit http://BonniesGang.com/

MATT AND PETER AND ELEMENT-X

I have two very good friends whom I have known for many years. They are both average-looking guys. Yet one of them was seeing four girls at one time with several more dates set up with different women and the other one has not had a successful date in years.

Let's call the guy seeing four girls at one time Matt and the guy with no game Peter. Matt actually ended up dumping a few of the girls he was dating because they eventually **disqualified** themselves (this is when a woman does not fit the criteria you are looking for, no matter how pretty she is or how good she is in bed).

Peter is 6 feet and 3 inches tall, which makes him an imposing figure, at least to the hottie who is only 5 feet, 6 inches tall. Matt on the other hand is 5 feet 9 inches tall and to most people looks like the average, well-dressed guy.

So, what is the difference between these two guys? Is it as simple as one guy has more natural ability to pick-up chicks than the other does? No way. One guy has Element-X and the other one wouldn't know it if it hit him in the ass.

I have been asking and researching the answers to these questions for years. Why is it that a guy like me, who used to suffer from panic attacks, was able to over come my shyness and begin having massive success with women? Why do Matt and Peter have different answers when I ask them *"how was your weekend bro?"*.

Matt: *My weekend was awesome. I went to a kick ass party Friday night with my date, Saturday morning I had dim sum with some friends, Saturday night I went dancing in Hollywood with another girl, and on Sunday, I watched football with my friends.*

Peter: *My weekend was ok. I played a lot of video games, didn't do much just hung around the house....my weekend blew man.*

Each time I ask my friends how their weekend went I usually get the same answer. One had a great weekend full of fun and **women** while the other one had either an "okay" weekend or one that "blew chunks".

Both guys have the same level of intelligence. Both of them have me as their friend (so you'd think having a dating coach as a friend would help right? Only if they listen). Both of them have access to the same level of information that I did when I started learning how to improve my game years ago. So, what is the difference? What's the one thing that separates the two?

The answer is that **it's not one thing.** Think of Element-X as a very delicious cake. When you take the cake out of the oven it's nearly done. All you have to do is add the frosting and whatever toppings you want on it. But to make that cake you need a bunch of other ingredients. The cake isn't made up of "cake"; it's made up of different things. That is what Element-X is like.

Once you know what the ingredients are, all you have to do is go to the super market, buy them, make the mix, put it in the oven, and bake that sucker.

Element-X is the same. You have to know what the ingredients are, put them into action, and then keep plugging away until it comes out right. Sometimes your first cake doesn't come out right, but your second cake will be a lot better (practice works!).

If you can view pick up or the ability to pick-up chicks in this manner it will be virtually impossible for you to fail. Getting good with the opposite sex is NOT a one-time event. Let me repeat that because this is very important to making this work.

You cannot view pick up as something that you do once, twice, or even a few times, it has to become a lifestyle change. Too many guys make the mistake of making a few approaches, it didn't turn the way they wanted, and then they think that:

1. *They are doomed to be single.*

2. *That what they learned does not work or it only works for other guys.*

I'm being dead serious when I ask you this: how much time would you give a baby to learn how to walk? Of course, the answer is *until they learn how to walk!*

I am not saying that you have to go make more than 100 approaches in one weekend. But before you start seeing some decent results like I did - you have got to view this whole game thing as a **process** and not a one-time event or something that you do a few times.

It takes some maturity and wisdom to understand this. Guess where maturity and wisdom comes from? That's right, it comes from **experience.** Some of the concepts in this report are not going to make any sense to you. Some of them will, but in order for you to really understand what I am talking about you have to get out there and experience these things for yourself.

For example, I can talk about using opinion openers all day long until I am blue in the face, but until you actually go out and make approaches you are not going to understand all the nuances that I talk about. Things such as girls giving one another eye signals, testing you, using your hand to tap them on the shoulder lightly but firmly enough to let them know that you're a man, and so on.

Element-X = That special something that a man has that women find attractive.

ELEMENT-X IS WAY MORE THAN CONFIDENCE

When I used to participate in seduction and pick up forums many guys would write *"all you need is confidence"* or *"you don't need advice, all you need is confidence".* That is easy to write when you already have it, but when you don't have it, it's very hard. I'm going to make it easier for you.

Let me ask you, have you ever been at a party, a club, or even just out and about in the public and notice some guy who is interacting with the opposite sex? He has them laughing and the women can't seem to get enough of him? Sometimes this guy is good-looking but generally, he is an average-looking guy.

Just like my friend Matt, he knows how to make himself appear above average **with his behavior**. Besides, most women respond far more to your personality than to your looks. I can't tell you how many of my ex-girlfriends and female friends have hooked up with troll-looking dudes just because of they way they acted.

A scientific fact that has been proven repeatedly. This is why it's very important to learn how to interact with women. You do this by working the system. It's just one style of pickup but it's very effective because women are biologically and psychologically wired to respond to certain things such as eye contact, body language, tone of voice, personality, confidence, style, humor, reality control, etc.

The Thing That Makes Element-X Work

If you were to ask 1,000 women what they like in a man they could never give you just "one" thing. They like cute butts, nice eyes, a man who can make them laugh, confidence in all things, leadership, gentleman, good in bed, great kisser, must "understand" her, etc. This holds true with Element-X. It takes a bunch of things to make it work.

One ingredient has to be there in order for Element-X to work. **Without this one thing, all the other ingredients that I'm going to share with you are meaningless!** This one thing I am about to share with you is what makes or breaks anyone who wants to try to improve their skill with women. It's what separates the men from the boys. It's also a huge reason why my friend Matt has 100 times more success with women than my friend Peter.

Here it is:

You have to change the way you view the real world in order to have more success with women.

Let it sink in for a minute. Now go back and re-read that last sentence because it's the first step to becoming good at your game....period! I'm not saying it's going to be easy. However, after reading this material you will be armed with the knowledge that will make it **easier than before.** That's a major distinction. In fact, once you finish reading this report you're going to know more about Element-X than 99% of the male population! My friend Peter thinks all women are evil, liars, and manipulative and it takes way *"too much work"* to get a date. With that perception of reality and women, it's no surprise that his ability to pick-up chicks sucks. It's the way he views reality that's causing him to blow chunks!

In contrast, my friend Matt thinks women are fascinating, interesting, and have to qualify for his time; that there's an abundance of them out there and there's always another woman around the corner if the one he's talking to or dating does meet up to his expectations. Matt and Peter have had very similar life experiences and I could make a case that Matt had a tougher childhood and life than Peter, yet Matt **chose to overcome any hurdle that came his way.**

So, what exactly do I mean that you have to change your view of the real world? Let me explain. Right now the way you perceive things are getting in the way of tightening your talent to pick-up hot women (think of my friend Peter and his view towards women).

It could be something as simple as thinking you're too short, too fat, too ugly, or as complicated as having issues with your parents. My friend Peter is miserable because he chooses to believe that all women are a certain way. That one perception of the real world is based on his life experience. Therefore, I don't fault him for believing that to a point. I do fault him for not trying to step outside of himself and taking an honest view of what this one belief is doing to his life. It's ruining his quality of life and not just with dating.

When I was a teenager, (a long time ago) I used to think that being 5 feet 5 inches tall really hurt me (I'm 5 inches taller today) and that girls only wanted guys to be over 6 feet tall. Isn't that what all the short girls write in their online profiles? I also used to believe that hot girls only dated hot guys. I also used to believe (or perceive) that hot girls only went out with guys with hot cars or kick-butt motorcycles.

I started questioning these false perceptions of reality when I met guys who weren't any better-looking than I was, shorter than I was, and didn't even own a car, yet they dated some hot girls. It blew my mind. I thought they probably had a lot of money. I was usually proven wrong. These guys had Element-X (that mystical "thing" that women find attractive).

It's also not as simple as **changing your belief system** (for more information on how to do this grab a paperback copy of Anthony Robbins AWAKEN THE GIANT WITHIN - this book drastically changed my life with women, my finances, my physical and mental health and is responsible for creating many millionaires, pick up artists, and many other successful people in all walks of life). Your belief system is part of Element-X, but only part of it (add another ingredient to your pick up cake).

When I say you have to change your perception of the real world I'm talking about making a conscious decision that you are going to try something new and commit to a plan of action no matter how fearful or uncertain you might be. *You cannot attain Element-X until you make this level of commitment to yourself!*

It's what my father used to call "being a man". A man takes 100% responsibility for his successes and failures. A real, mature man does not blame others or circumstances for his problems - even if it's true! When I stopped blaming my looks, my height, and other people for the problems in my life, my life started improving on all levels. I started eating better. I created a budget. I exercised more often. I eliminated the word "rejection" from my vocabulary. I made a commitment to my own personal growth and began making approaches even though I knew I was going to make a ton of mistakes and be blown out. Yes, I realize this might sound cheesy, but cheesy works sometimes. I'm not going to reinvent decades of research. Instead of fighting it, I decided to come on board and change my life, no matter what.

That's probably not the answer you were looking for, but my job here is to share with you what works, not what you want to hear. I've received thousands of e-mails, phone calls, IMs, text messages, and even snail mail from men around the world telling me that what they learned worked for them once they put it into practice. I didn't invent Element-X.

Element-X has worked for thousands of years. Every single person has the ability to learn how to get it, if they're willing to work for it. So, the first step to making Element-X work for you is to spend a day or a weekend away from your family, friends, etc. and spend some time seriously thinking how badly you want to succeed with women.

To take it further, think about how you want to succeed in life. Whatever that means to you. **Hint:** *Women are attracted to men who **know** where they are going in life because women are very future-orientated. It is also a higher status quality.*

I used to think that success meant having a girlfriend (a lot of guys think this way, pick up artists think the opposite). Now I know that kind of thinking is wrong. When people are on their deathbed they usually want to be surrounded by people they love. No one on their deathbed wishes they had spent more time at the office, worked on the yard more, had a bigger home, watched more TV, a nicer car, or had a girlfriend, etc. We'll talk more about that later. Remember, if you're not willing to change the way you think, then the rest of this report will not do you any good. At least keep an open mind about it for now. You should re-read this report at least a few times a year to help you keep your focus.

The next logical question is "*ok Jani, that's fine and dandy, but* **how** *do I go about doing this? How do I change the way I think?*"

Well, I already gave you the first step and that was to make a decision that you deserve better, which means you're willing to do the work necessary to change the way you think.

The following step is that you have to **write it down**. I'm not going to go into all the studies that have proven that writing down something helps in a big way, all you have to understand at this point is that if you don't write it down then you haven't really made a commitment yet (one study has shown that writing down something increases your chances at achieving it by ten times!). Then reviewing it daily increases the odds tremendously. Want to

134

know what I first wrote down years ago? Here it is:

I'm going to go out on a date with a gorgeous girl within one year.

This doesn't have to be your first goal. I'm just sharing mine years ago when I had no ability to pick-up hot women and had to give my mind something to focus on. Notice how I gave myself a whole year to do this, there's no sense in putting more pressure on yourself than you have to. The important thing is that I wrote it down and I reviewed it every day. Let's take all the emotion out of this goal and focus on the logical sequence for a minute. In order for me to eventually reach my goal of going out on a date with a hot girl within a 365-day period, I knew that I had to talk to many girls. When you break it down day-by-day, it's actually not a whole lot.

The thought of approaching girls I didn't know terrified me back then. As a man, I hate to admit that, but it's the truth. Today I still get a little nervous every now and then, but women in and of them don't scare me anymore. The same thing can happen to you with enough practice.

I am going to repeat that repeatedly because it's that important. I couldn't picture myself walking up to a stranger that I didn't even know. On top of my extreme shyness, I also suffered from panic attacks, which made my young adult years really tough on me. But I knew that if I didn't do anything nothing would happen. Just like the saying goes:

If you do the same things every day then the next 5 years will be just like your last 5 years. Is this something you really want?

So I grit my teeth, went to the library and devoured every book about dating, kissing, and affairs that I could get my hands on (something I don't necessarily recommend because today you've got the Internet, but back in the day there wasn't any Internet). Most of them were off the mark, but at least I did learn a few things. For the next couple of weekends I went to as many different night clubs that my time and wallet could afford. All I did was walk around and observed how men and women interacted. I had never done that before. I learned a lot from just watching. I even had a few girls walk up to me, but I really didn't have much to say. Believe it or not, knowing that I was only there to watch and observe helped me relax. There was no pressure to perform.

Before I knew it a few months had passed and I didn't even have one date set up. I was really frustrated. So I did something that was way outside my **comfort zone**. I went to an amusement park with my friends and began walking up to nearly every girl I saw. I ended up approaching over 60 girls in one day! I bombed most of them because I was so shy, but I had reached the point where I did not care. I had to learn how to overcome my shyness, even though my hands shook so badly that I had to put them in my pockets!

Then, the next day I went to another amusement park and by the end of the weekend I had walked up to over 100 girls. I was a lot better at my 100th approach then my first. I'm talking by a mile. I was way better at approaching girls by the end of the weekend. I felt like I had crammed years of learning into one weekend.

Think about it for a minute. If I only approached 2 or 3 girls a year I just completed decades worth of approaching in that one weekend. There were several times where I actually had fun walking up to groups of girls because I had no idea what would happen. Today I still have this passion. I still don't know what will happen, though I'm far better at reading body language now and have gotten much better at predicting outcomes. But the outcome isn't something you should care about.

Now don't freak out on me. I'm not saying you have to do this. I just want to illustrate that writing down a goal is paramount to attaining Element-X. I wrote down my goal and went about it in a way that I thought was the best way at the time. Well, after making 100 approaches in one weekend I realized I had made a big mistake. I forgot to ask the girls for their phone numbers! For a moment I got really bummed out because I felt like my whole weekend went to waste. But remembering my commitment to going for it I realized that I had overcome a huge chunk of my shyness. So I began feeling better.

I began approaching girls at the mall, bowling alleys, the super market, on the street, in music stores, book stores, bagel shops, carnivals, parties, and if you can name a public place I probably asked a girl for her phone number there. I even talked to girls after church services!

I was serious about meeting my goal of seeing on a regular basis a gorgeous girl within 365 days. It took me nearly a year, but after going out with a few trolls, a couple of self-centered bitches, I finally met a hot girl who agreed to go out on a date with me and ended up liking me. I had met my first goal. But my work had just begun. I didn't just want to date one hot girl. I wanted to get good at pick up. I wanted Element-X to become part of who I was, not something that was mechanical and contrived.

In order for that to happen I knew I had to continue making approaches, making mistakes, and dating different kinds of women.

RAISE YOUR GROUP VALUE

Women are attracted to men with high group value. Put another way women are not attracted to losers (unless they have their own issues, but that's an entirely different report that won't do you any good). In my eyes my friend Peter is not a loser because I've known him for years. The guy is my brother from another mother. This is why you need to have the discipline to take all your feelings away from any situation and look at it with a fresh pair of eyes.

But to be totally frank, if I had just met Peter today I would probably think he was a loser. He complains a lot. He still dresses the same way he did in high school and college. He has a slouch, which he can easily correct (slouching conveys low status). He plays over 30 hours of video games per week. He rarely leaves his home. He lives on fast food and his beer belly gets a little bigger every year. Like I said, I love the guy, but if he doesn't change the way he perceives reality he's going to be a lonely, grumpy old man. **Remember that you cannot change another person, they have to want to change** (this advice will save you from marrying the wrong woman). I give him advice when he asks, but he's so set in his ways I might as well be talking to the wall.

Here's the scary part. Peter views himself as having high group value because he has a high IQ, a very good job, and feels like he is a "good man". The problem with this way of thinking is that it's not based on the real world. The majority of attractive woman would rate confidence over IQ any day of the week. Most women would prefer a man who knows how to flirt than a man who is smart. Peter's ever-growing beer belly is also a huge sign of low group value because it communicates to women *"I don't have any respect for myself"*. Men with high group value take care of their bodies, their hair, their hygiene, and value their health.

Attractive women in our society have built-in high group value. They don't have to lift a finger, which is why they generally have an "entitlement" mentality. Men fawn over them, other women hate them, and they are used to getting what they want. Attractive men also have built-in higher group value, but it's only 1/10th of attractive women because **men are far more visual than women are**.

I can't tell you how many attractive men have sought out the services of a dating coach because their looks weren't enough. You have to have *some* talent to pick-up hot women. If you are shy and can't talk to women then how can you ever get their digits, let alone a date with them? Rich men with no game attempt to impress women with expensive gifts, exotic vacations to far away places, their job or business, or some other form of materialism. Not the thing to do … bad move.

You obtain some group value by being rich, famous, handsome, or having a personality that creates attraction. While there are many new millionaires being created every single day, we're not going to focus on this. Let's focus on things you have more control over. What I'm about to share with you isn't rocket science and you probably already know this on an intellectual level. But until you make it hit your emotional gut, nothing will happen. You can start creating higher group value as soon as today. So let's get to it!

What Does Your Physical Appearance Say About You?

Let's face it, men who look fit and healthy have higher group value then men with beer bellies or who are visibly out of shape. I used to be like Peter, eating fast food for breakfast, lunch, and dinner. In one year I managed to gain more than 50 pounds. No wonder the cute girls wouldn't talk to me. Women may not be as visual as men are but it doesn't take much to turn them off either.

So I stopped eating junk food, stopped stocking my fridge with beer and soda, and began eating foods that I freaking hated like broccoli, cabbage, lettuce, spinach, and I even got a juicer and drank fresh juice. After a few weeks I felt so much better that I actually began liking broccoli, fish, baked chicken without the skin, rare red meat, ate only healthy oils like coconut oil and olive oil -- and even drastically cut down on grains and sugars. Yeah, go figure.

This totally changed my life (far more than I expected)**.** I slept better, I felt better, and I had more mental clarity which helped me at work, with my group skills, and even my sex life. If that doesn't convince you to eat better then I don't know what will. Look at the rapper 50 Cent. He got buffed out by doing a lot of sit ups and push ups virtually every day. So you don't need any fancy gym equipment or memberships. All you need to do is take a visit to your medical professional so they can give you the thumbs up and then the discipline to see it through. Always get a thorough physical before you start any kind of work out program, no matter how old you are.

That's how I got buffed out. When I'm at a party or night club I almost always have some girl tell me I have "nice arms". That leaves them open for a witty remark like *"yeah, take a number"* or *"if I had a dime for every time I heard that"* or *"listen, just say you like me, I know I have sexy arms"* or *"What? How can you **not** see my sexy ear lobes?"*.

You have total control over what you put in your mouth, so start eating better, start going for walks, take the stairs instead of the elevator, and take up some form of exercise that you can't get out of. For example, I've had students take dancing classes, swimming lessons, tennis lessons, join a basketball league.....whatever got them to get moving at least 3 to 4 times a week for 30 minutes at a time. Just make sure you see your physician before you join any kind of physical program.

Men who know how to dress also have a perceived higher group value. My sense of style has improved over the years, but I'm far from a fashion guru. As of this writing I own 4 pairs of jeans (one of them is a designer label, but you don't need that), about a dozen shirts that I can wear for going out, a handful of t-shirts with witty comments in the front or back (plus, I love Harleys, so a fair share of black Harley type t-shirts) , a couple of suits, 2 leather jackets, 2 "cool-looking" jackets that women picked out for me, some slacks, 4 belts, and about 4 pairs of shoes and 2 pairs of sneakers. That's a tiny ass wardrobe compared to the women I've dated. Yet I get complimented on how I dress all the time.

Here's the kicker: the women in my life have picked out most of my clothes. Women I've dated, my sisters, my female friends, or the good-looking sales clerk who is paid to be nice. At the very least I don't like to go shopping for clothes or shoes without a stylish female. I'm no fashion expert, but one thing I do know about is good shoes. I like them in black leather - casual and fancy. In the warm months, there is nothing wrong with flip-flops. You don't have to go high end to look good.

The majority of women like how I dress, but hey, you can't impress them all. That's not your goal anyway. Your goal is not to impress. Your goal is to look good for yourself and to be comfortable. Wearing cutoff jean shorts and a tank top at most venues is neither looking good, nor all that comfortable and it screams of low group value.

When you are picking a style of dress for yourself, you want to wear something that you're comfortable in, look good on you and communicates that you give a damn about what you look like. I've got my own style and it's actually quite conservative compared to some of the other dating coaches and pick up artists I've met in the field. But it works for me. That's the key. It has to work for you.

Go shopping with a sister, cousin, or female friend who understands style. If you don't have any of those find a store that has an attractive female clerk and ask her honest opinion on what would look good on you for going out, casual dinners, or just opening your door when someone knocks on it. You'll be pleasantly surprised at how helpful most of them will be. Here's what I love to do when I go shopping for clothes when none of my girlfriends are available. I'll find a cute clerk and ask her to help me pick out an outfit, but using some form of role-play (women love role-playing, at least the ones that are fun):

Me: Hi, I'm looking to buy a new outfit for clubbing. So how's your fashion sense? (I've never heard a hot female clerk say, "I suck").

Her: It's pretty good.

Me: Only pretty good? C'mon.....

Her: Well, I don't want to sound like I'm bragging.

Me: Ah, brag away, it's healthy.

Her: (Giggle).

Me: Ok, pretend that you're my girlfriend and that tonight we're going to a very trendy nightclub where celebrities hang out. Point me in the right direction.

Her: I can do that, though my boyfriend wouldn't like that.

Me: (Never show women that you're fazed by their comments) Ha ha! That's funny, he's not here.....besides it's only make believe. My girlfriend wouldn't mind, in fact she'd go with it. Ok now, pick out an outfit that would look good on me.

Her: This could be fun.

Me: I'm always a load of fun. By the way, my name is Jani.

Her: Alea.

Me: Cool name. Ok now, let's take a look over here.......

      If you take this tactic when shopping for clothes or shoes, you'll get a lot of excellent feedback from clerks whose job it is to help you. Every once in a while, I'll run into a cute female clerk who is having a bad day. For whatever reason she is not motivated to help me. If I'm in no real hurry, I'll attempt to turn her mood around by saying *"Hey, I'm a very intuitive person and my intuition tells me that you're normally smiling and happy. So I've got to ask, what's the matter?"*

      Now tone of voice communicates a lot so you don't want to ask this like a wimp, but in a firm, but friendly voice. If you're normally soft spoken, make it a point to speak a couple decibels louder than you normally talk. Remember that there's background noise in most public places and you should be talking louder than normal anyway. Okay, back to fashion.

      My friend Matt likes to wear suits, slacks, cuff links, and blazers. That works for him. I'm more of a jeans, nice collared, pressed shirt with leather shoes type of guy. Peter likes to wear plain polo shirts or t-shirts with nerdy stuff on them (think Weird Al, World of Warcraft, comic book characters, cartoons, etc.) and he always tucks in his shirt with his belt (does not always look cool tucking shirts that are not meant to be tucked). His beer / fast food belly sticks out and screams of lower group value and no self-respect for himself. If all Peter did was buy a few cooler shirts, lost the beer belly, improved his posture, he'd be much better off. Even so, he still wouldn't be close to attaining Element-X because he hasn't changed the way he perceives reality and that's what makes Element-X work.

Yellow teeth can be whitened, dandruff can be controlled, moles and crappy tattoos can be lasered off, acne can be controlled or eliminated, weight can be controlled, bad breath can be eliminated, ear / nose / back hair can be waxed / lasered / shaved off. Make a list right now of the physical things in your control. If you don't write it down you'll never change them. So, write them down and form a plan to get them taken care of.

I once had a student who didn't believe in using breath mints, changing his underwear every day, and didn't think using deodorant was important (I'm not kidding!). No wonder he didn't get any dates, his body odor scared the women away. Women have very sensitive noses, which is why personal hygiene is crucial. It's also another reason why you don't need a lot of cologne. One or two sprays in the air before you put your clothes on and walking through the mist right after you spray it is more than good enough.

REALITY CONTROL

"Whoever controls their own reality controls their own situation." -
-Anonymous

The following concept has many different names; it has been called frame control, paradigm, shifting, etc. No matter what name you give it, this is so powerful that dictators have been able to control the minds of millions using it. The most common reason - other than doing nothing - why men fail with women is that **they allow the woman to control their perception of the real world**, which means they are allowing her to control the situation or at least the perception of it. All right, so you really can't control actual reality, but **you can control how you perceive and react to the real world.** That's where the real power lies.

Therefore, when some girl tells me *"I have a boyfriend"* the old me would allow her to control my perception of the real world and I would say *"okay"* and then walk away. Today I might say something like *"really, that's cool how did you two meet?"* or *"that's cool, I'm glad we got that out of the way"* and then I would continue talking since half the time they really don't have a boyfriend anyway. Continuing to talk when she tries to blow you off is very powerful. You should try it sometime soon.

You have control over your reality to a much higher degree than you think. My reality today is that I'm such a cool, likable guy that any woman who doesn't want to interact with me probably has a corkscrew loose in her head. She might be having a bad night. She might be a man-hater. More than one rude man might have approached her before I walked up to her. No matter what, there's something going on with her and it's not me because I already know I'm a cool guy. That's my reality and nothing a woman says or does can change that. It took me months to really believe that, but man, it was worth all the hard work.

Let me ask you a question. Do you have more respect for a man who tries and fails or a man who never tries? Of course, we respect the man who at least tries.

When I walk up to a woman in a super market and there are people around, I'm not thinking about what she thinks of me or what the people around think of me. I'm not allowing the situation to control my perception of my reality. Men who have Element-X know all about this.

The man with Element-X will approach this attractive woman thinking that he's giving her a great opportunity to meet him. The man without Element-X will approach this woman thinking that she might think he's weird, that she might reject him, and that the people around them are going to think he's a pervert or some horny dude.

See the difference? Neither real world is true, yet you make it true by the way you interpret it.

You can use reality control in your everyday life, not just in pick up. You can use it to feel happier, have more energy, attain motivation, and a whole bunch of other things. Think of my two friends Matt and Peter, who do you think has more control over their own perception of the real world? Matt clearly believes he has more control, while Peter believes other forces have more control.

In my old wuss days, if I walked up to girl at a nightclub and asked her to dance I would interpret her answer of "no" as rejection. I allowed it to ruin my whole night. When I got four "no's" in a row I believed that I was a loser. But in reality, I wasn't a loser because at least I tried. A loser is someone who never tries or quits on trying. Today when I ask a girl to dance and she says "no" I like to have fun with it. Here's a recent example of how I controlled my own reality and therefore my own situation:

Me: Hey, this song rocks, let's dance.

Her: Sorry, I'm tired.

Me: Tired? That's funny you don't look tired (smirk).

Her: Well, I'm really tired.

Me: You're right. I realize that I'm asking you to dance to one or two songs, but I can see why you're tired. We'll dance, you'll see my mad dance skills, fall in love with me, we'll get married, and then you'll discover that I squeeze the toothpaste from the middle of the tube and then we'll get divorced. You're right you shouldn't dance with me. I can see where this is going because all I want to do is dance to a couple of songs. I don't want you to know that I squeeze toothpaste from the middle of the tube.

Her: You're a weird one (trying not to smile).

Me: Yeah, but in a good way (rephrase her attempt of knocking you down by spinning it into a positive way). Tell you what, after two songs I'll return you back to your friends in one piece as long as you promise not to fall in love with me. I have enough people stalking me these days (said while extending my hand out and looking her right in the eye).

Her: Ok, I guess it can't hurt.

Even if she didn't dance with me, I would still be having a good time because I have to have some fun with someone who gave me a ridiculous answer. It's a ridiculous answer because women are rarely "tired" when they go to nightclubs, especially if it isn't even midnight yet.

I want you to notice in the example how I rephrased and controlled my perception of the real world while demonstrating Element-X. Notice how I did not buy her excuse of being tired. Men let women get off the hook too easily these days. I like to challenge them a bit. Sure, she might have been tired, but chances are it was her pat answer that she uses all the time. So to get over that I wanted to persist without being a jerk. She doesn't know it but I'm also testing her to see if she's even worth my time. So, a girl who doesn't want to dance with me isn't worth my time anyway. In my world, the party is wherever I go. That's reality control baby!

The Most Important Person In The World

People with a healthy dose of high self-esteem do not allow outside things affect how they feel about themselves in the long-term. If my friends Matt and Peter were to walk up to a woman to ask her out and she said *"no"*, my friend Matt would shrug his shoulders, wish her a nice day, and move on. One minute later, he has already forgotten about the small interaction. Peter, also hearing the "no" would probably bug her and ask her "why not?" and then would go home, sit on his couch and stew about it all day long.

To make Element-X become part of who you are **you have to believe you are the most important person in your world**. I'm not talking about becoming a narcissistic, self-

152

centered jerk because that's not healthy. I'm talking about a healthy idea in your mind that no hot woman is more important than yourself and your own happiness. Now that's real power.

Have you ever met a man who was cocky, arrogant, and seemed to have a lot of confidence? I'm sure you have; now that's not what I'm talking about. Men like that are actually insecure people and they mask their insecurities by acting cocky and arrogant. Most people they meet view them as self-centered jerks; for good reason, they are. Sure, they might attract some women, but these women generally have issues. Healthy, mature, fun women with self-esteem are not attracted to these kinds of men.

I'm not talking about arrogance or cockiness here; I'm talking about putting yourself first. It's this simple: men who do not have Element-X usually put women first in their interactions, whereas men with Element-X usually put themselves first in their interactions with women. Let me give you some examples of what I'm talking about. This holds true in approaching, dating, and even in relationships to a certain extent.

The Girl With "Standards"

I was set to go on a date with a girl named Ashley. I had already screened her on an online personal ad, then over the phone, and only then did I decide we should meet up person. Going out to dinners and expensive dates are a waste of time and money when you're going to go on a first time date (I call these "first meetings" and not dates). I like to meet women for drinks at coffee shops, malls (walking around does wonders for getting to know someone), restaurant bars, etc. I like giving women options so I asked Ashley if she wanted to meet up for drinks at XYZ coffee shop or go to the mall and do some window-shopping.

She didn't want to do either. She suggested that we have dinner at this fine Italian restaurant in Beverly Hills (I never go to a fine dining establishment with someone I have not dated for awhile). I don't date women to impress them or to cater to them. All I'm doing in the beginning is trying to screen out the flakes, gold diggers, phonies, etc. Since I'm the most important person in my world and I know exactly what I want, I told her politely that I did not want to go out to dinner. I first wanted to grab a drink or go for a walk somewhere so we could talk. She would not budge. She wanted to go out and eat. She tried to explain to me that she had certain "tastes" and "standards" and believed in going out to dinner for the purposes of getting to know someone (could you smell the crap coming out of that answer?).

In reality, all she really wanted was a free meal. I don't date women who have ridiculous "standards" or certain "tastes" which is why I never give into ultimatums or unreasonable preferences. So in the situation, who was more important? Ashley or me (meaning my wallet)? I decided to choose me and told her that when and if she wanted to meet up for drinks to give me a call. That was the end of that. Ashley never called me. This was fine with me, because I was already setting up other first meetings with other women (another reason why you should never focus on only one woman at a time).

THE NEW CAR WITH A SHINY RED RIBBON

Robert was a successful attorney in Los Angeles. At age 34 he had his own successful practice and also owned another business. I met Robert at a mixer and he shared a funny story with me. Robert had Element-X. Here's what happened to him. He met a 26 year old model named Barbara. She was gorgeous, tall, and every man wanted her. Robert met her through a mutual friend and they began seeing each other.

After a couple months of dating, Barbara and Robert were having dinner at a cool Indian Restaurant when she asked him for something out of the ordinary. This is how the conversation went and I'm proud to say that Robert held his ground by choosing himself first:

Barbara: I can't believe I'm going to be 27 soon.

Robert: At least you're not turning 30.

Barbara: You're right. You want to hear something cool?

Robert: I'm always down for "cool", let's hear it.

Barbara: Well, my sisters had been seeing her boyfriend Brad for almost a year and guess what he got her for her birthday?

Robert: I have no idea; I'm not sure what your sister likes. But I'll bite. He bought her flowers and took her to a nice place with a view for dinner.

Barbara: No silly, he bought her a car! And it was so cute! He even put a red ribbon around it.

Robert: Wow, that guy is crazy!

Barbara: Why is he crazy? I think it's romantic.

Robert: No, watching a sunset together is romantic, buying someone a car who isn't your wife is just plain lunacy.

Barbara: So if I wanted a car for my birthday you wouldn't buy me one?

Robert: You're kidding right?

Barbara: What is wrong with asking for a car?

Robert: Wow, I've never seen this side of you.

Barbara: What side? Because I'm asking for a car?

Robert: Exactly. I might buy a family member a car if they really needed it or my spouse if I had one......

Barbara: Other men have offered to buy me a car.

Robert: (Incredulous) Great, then you should date those other men.

Barbara: I can't believe you wouldn't buy someone you love a car.

Robert: Woah, woah....I never said I loved you.

Barbara: Whattttt!!!!!!

So an argument ensued, but Robert didn't budge. He asked for the bill, dropped Barbara off at her place, and broke up with her. Why? Because Robert put himself first. He knows there are other women, though some women act as if they are the last females on earth.

You might be surprised at how many men buy women things like cars, homes, expensive jewelry, dinners, just to keep them around and to keep them happy (ridiculous). Robert put himself first and would not cater to a woman's "high standards". Within a couple of weeks he was already seeing someone just as attractive and she never asked him for a car.

I'm using the "car" as an example of the extreme. More often than not, it will be her asking for expensive dates or to take her shopping.

"I Hate That Song"

I love music. All kinds. I play it in my car, in my room, in my house, and on my MP3 player. Every once in a while some woman will say *"I hate that song"* or *"I hate that kind of music."* My response is usually *"well, I like it and that's all that matters."* If we're in **my** home or car, I never turn it off because I want to listen to it. She has the option of going to another room or simply putting up with it. If it becomes an issue then I'd have to spell it out to her that I would never presume to tell her what to do in her own home or car. You're the king of your castle, which means where you live, inside your car, etc. The music you listen to should never be an issue, but with some women, they try to make it one. I also make it a point to indirectly tell women with my responses one or two things:

1. No one is more important than I am.

2. There is always another woman that I can find who won't act this way.

"I Would Never Go Out With You"

158

When I was a wuss I heard this from time to time when I would ask a girl for her phone number. Today I rarely hear it because I have Element-X. When you approach a woman, you're going to hear a variety of responses and most of the time you'll find that women are actually cool as long as you're not creepy.

The first time I heard a woman tell me she would never go out with me I was very crushed. This made no sense because she was a stranger and didn't really know me. It's interesting how we are quick to interpret a woman's response as "rejection" when nothing could be further from the truth. **Only people that know you and care about can reject you.**

Today if a woman were to ever say, *"I would never go out with you"* if I wanted to be mean I could simply reply with *"no biggie, there's someone else younger and hotter than you that will."* In addition, I'd simply walk away. But that's not my style, I usually just say *"Great! Have a awesome week!"* I walk away and forget about the whole thing. There's zero benefit to holding onto the past. She's already forgotten about you, why not pay her the same favor?

Remember that no one is more important than you are when it comes to meeting and dating women. You don't have to be a complete asshole jerk when you say these things. I even say them with a smirk or a wink sometimes, but I'm firm and I make eye contact. No matter what a woman says to you, it's not personal, so don't make it something it's not. There's always another girl around the corner. Always.

KNOW WHAT YOU WANT!

Another Element-X ingredient is **knowing what you want.** Once you know what you want, write it down. Imagine the power you will have when you know what you want and nothing will distract you from getting it. I've seen too many men make major changes in their lives when they didn't want to or when they were not ready for it simply because a woman asked them to.

I've had many girlfriends ask me to move in with them or to move in with me. One even asked me only after one month of seeing her! Talk about a major red flag! My answer today is always *"no"* because I do not believe in living together (my own personal choice).

Some women also like to give ultimatums.

"If you don't marry me I'm leaving!"

"If you don't buy me a ring, we're through!"

"You're cheap because you didn't spend enough money on me!"

*"If we don't go to ***** this summer I'm going to go with someone else."*

"If you watch football this Sunday I'm going to..."

When a man knows exactly what he wants in life, it's far easier to control his own reality. When you know what you want you will not give into unreasonable ultimatums. A few years ago, I was at a rock concert with my girlfriend at the time. About an hour into it, everyone in the stadium was on their feet, dancing away and having a good time.

Now my girlfriend and I had been together for 3 years, so it was a serious relationship. I noticed she wasn't having a good time so I asked her what the deal was. She said she was tired and that she wanted go.

Here's some background: I had told her that before we went to the concert that we were going to watch the whole show, which would have lasted about 2 hours. It's important to set expectations early on.

Well this young woman already knew what I was like and already knew my expectations so I suspected she wanted to pick a fight or there was some other issue going on that she didn't want to bring up (most women are VERY indirect). I told her she could go relax at the lounge outside and that I would meet up with her there. I even offered to check up on her from time to time.

She would not have it. She began to pout and complain, knowing full well this was one of my favorite bands and that I had been looking forward to it all year long. She made a big mistake: she gave me the unreasonable ultimatum:

Her: *If we don't leave right now I'm going to call a taxi.*

Me: *Go ahead.*

Her: *If you let me go home in cab, we're through!*

Me: *Well, I never thought you would ever throw down a selfish ultimatum. Go ahead and call your cab. Then I want you to spend the next few days thinking about if our positions were reversed how would you want me to act. Later.*

So, she called her cab and left. Even though we had been together for 3 years, she finally decided to show her true self. One thing I don't do when I'm dating women or in a relationship with women is to spend energy on figuring out why they are doing something or WHY they do certain things. In the example I just gave you she could have wanted to break up and this was her way of getting out. She could have had a lousy day and chose not to share that with me - my point here is that my focus was to enjoy the concert as I had planned and not waste energy on why my girlfriend (now ex-girlfriend) chose to be immature and selfish. I not only had a great time at the concert, I walked away with a couple of phone numbers from girls that I ran into while I walked around (some venues are simply awesome for walking around and meeting girls).

This is another reason why I don't believe in short engagements (if you're planning on getting married). You really don't know someone until you've seen him or her under duress. When I didn't call her after a couple of weeks she finally called me wondering if we really were through. I told her I was already dating two other women and thanked her for being selfish that night. She wanted to remain friends, but I had so many female friends already that I didn't want another one, at least not her.

This is how powerful this concept is: **you have to know what you want** because it will help you hold your ground during the really tough times. You will also know how to deal with selfish ultimatums. Just because I was with her for 3 years didn't mean that she now had free reign to act like a selfish person. Some women get sulky when they are not the center of attention.

Looking back on that relationship we shouldn't have lasted 3 years anyway. I was a younger man back then. This is why I'm **not** a big believer in dating only a few women and then settling down because the more women you date, the wiser you will get and you'll have a much clearer idea on what you want. If I had my way, every man would have to date at least 99 women before they ever got married (and I suspect that the divorce rate would go down by half!).

I'll tell you right now. What I thought I wanted when I was 18 years old changed quite a bit when I turned 25. When I turned 30, it was very different because I had already gone on over 150 dates and I exposed myself to a wide variety of women. Once you have tight game and you know you can get a woman anytime you want, you WILL not put up with crap behavior.

You might not know exactly what you want right now, but you should write down what you think you want. Ever heard of a movie called WEIRD SCIENCE? It's about these two unpopular, dorky high school guys who thought all they needed in life was a hot woman. So they discovered a way to use their computer to create what they thought was the perfect woman. Since these two guys had never had much experience with the opposite sex, they didn't really know what they wanted.

Ultimately, they woman that they created put them through many tough challenges. **She pushed these two guys outside their comfort zones.** By putting them in tough situations, they began to have new experiences, including with the opposite sex. By the time the movie ended, both of these guys had more self-confidence and had a clearer idea on what they wanted. They ended up telling the perfect woman that they still loved her but had hooked up with these two cute, popular girls. The woman, named Lisa, told them that even though she was hurt, all she wanted for them was to be happy and confident.

The more you push yourself outside your comfort zone (i.e. approaching women, going out on dates, seeing a variety of women, etc.) the better idea you will get on what you want in a woman. Today I know exactly what I want in a woman and I'm sure it's going to continue to evolve and change. This allows me to weed out the kinds of girls I don't want in my life. They've got to adapt and adjust to my life, not the other way around. You'll be able to be fussy too if you really apply yourself. You'll be shocked how different your life can change in 3 to 5 months if you really stick to it.

HOW TO BECOME POWERFUL

Men who have Element-X are powerful men. By it's very definition any man who has Element-X is powerful. The dictionary defines power as follows: *ability to do or act; capability of doing or accomplishing something.* Power means the ability to do something. If you want to become more successful with women, you have to take action (which makes you powerful). That's another ingredient in how to obtain Element-X. You cannot attain it by sitting down and reading this report. You have to formulate a plan of action and do it.

No two women are alike on this planet, but they all can sense when a male is powerful. They know the difference between a man who does NOT take action to one that does. When you have the following ingredients women will either be attracted to you or, at the very least, have respect for you.

I did not overcome my shyness by staying at home or hiding behind my homework or my career. I overcame it by having these ingredients and taking massive action. I have listed them here in no particular order:

1. Reality Control

2. Changing perception of the real world (for example, changing what "rejection" means).

3. Writing down goals.

4. Raising group value (for example, taking control of your physical body, fashion sense, communicating to women that you have a life).

5. Knowing that you are the most important person when it comes to dealing with or having relationships with women (too many men put attractive women on a pedestal, you should treat

them as equals - it's more fun to treat them as though they were your little sister).

6. Know what you want (too often I've heard men say "I'd just be happy with a girlfriend" and that's such a powerless statement to make because it means that they are willing to settle for any woman that will like them or give them a chance).

7. Become powerful by taking action.

Here's something you have to realize. You **must** use all seven of these ingredients to obtain Element-X. Having one, two, or even four out of the seven will NOT do it. By knowing these seven ingredients and combining them, you'll create such an unstoppable force that you'll be able to attain Element-X in a 3 to 5 month period. How can I be so certain? I've seen it hundreds of times in men all around the world, not just my country.

A man who has Element-X is powerful by definition because he has taken consistent and massive action. This is how you become powerful. Here are some examples on how some of my friends and many of my students gained power by attaining Element-X:

Brian, 19 years old
"Yo Jani, I stopped eating fast food, started drinking water instead of soda and I followed your advice about walking everyday. It has been

2 months and I have already lost 33 pounds! Thanks bro!"

Billy, 33 years old

"I sucked at dating. In my whole life I only had two girlfriends and they were both nasty. I was a loser with a capital L. I finally grew a pair and decided to write down that I would kiss the hottest girl at the local nightclub before the year ended (I had 4 months left). You advised me not to go to that club but to go to other clubs in a different city. So I spent a month or so working on my craft. I walked up to girls at clubs, at bars, at malls, and I struck gold when I went on Match.com.

It was kind of pricey but I set up a few dates. My confidence really began to grow Jani. I was turned down a lot during the first month or so but at month number two, I walked up to this hot girl. She was a college student at San Diego State, I grabbed her by the hand after a few minutes, and we ended up making out in the patio. I'm kicking ass and taking names!"

Devon, 24 years old

"Dude, you're going to think I'm crazy. I wrote down that I would approach 100 girls in one weekend like you did. I crashed two parties that weekend, then I went to a rave and I approached over 112 girls. Some of them were somewhat chubby but some of them were hot. I got more than 10 phone numbers...but I don't even care about that. I'm a changed man forever thanks to you."

Melissa, 21 years old

"Hi!!!!! I know I'm a girl but want to thank you because you totally saved me! I've been reading your newsletter (is that what it's called?) for over a year and you inspired me to lose weight and pay attention to what guys liked. I have the best boyfriend in the world now thanks to you. I totally controlled my reality. I've lost 22 pounds and now all the men won't leave me alone."

Nick, 42

"I've only been in the US for a little while and have always wanted to date a pretty blond woman, but my attempts have always ended in failure. I decided to follow your advice and changed the way I dressed. I also focused less on getting a blond woman and focused more on practicing my group skills. I talked louder than I was used to and practiced looking at women in the eyes when I talked to them. This was very difficult for me because of my thick accent. I joined Toastmasters like you advised and it really helped with my confidence. I strongly recommend it for anyone who is shy or has issues with public speaking.

I made many approaches and met with failure upon failure. But I always remembered that power equals action. I could only fail if I stopped trying. After several months, I began learning the subtleties of the English language. I was beginning to understand what 'cool' meant. I thought it was an immature and meaningless term, but I realized that being 'cool' had to do with group status and nothing to do with what I thought it was.

I began obtaining more phone numbers, mostly using the Internet. I met some crazy women. I also met some nice ones. I am currently seeing a pretty blond woman. Thank you for your help."

You may be wondering if Matt and Peter really exist; yes, they do. They are both good friends of mine, yet they have both chosen very two different group and life paths. Element-X isn't just some gimmicky name. It's not just a word. It's a way of thinking and a way of life.

Once it becomes part of who you are, you'll never get bothered if something doesn't go your way. As fate would have it, my friend Matt is visiting with me today as I was typing up this section and he walked into my room to say "goodbye".

He told me that his date for tonight had flaked on him. I asked him if he was bummed out (I should know by now to not ask him this question). He replied and said "no" and that he had already made a few phone calls and was going to go out with some other girl.

Matt has Element-X, which means he is powerful because he was willing to take action. Matt rarely eats junk food while Peter eats nothing but junk food. Matt drinks about two sodas a week (usually Coke Zero) while Peter drinks 3 to 5 sodas a day. Matt consistently approaches 10 to 15 girls a week, though he's so good at it now he doesn't really need to approach that many. Peter approaches 1 to 2 girls per year.

Matt exercises 3 to 4 times a week. Peter thinks exercising means playing World of Warcraft for hours at a time. Matt has six very close friends in his inner circle, roughly 225 professional contacts, and over 50 acquaintances.

Peter has two close friends, roughly five or six professional contacts, and a handful of acquaintances. Matt focuses on living in the now. Peter complains about the past and about all the wrongs that people have done to him over the years.

Matt loves meeting new people. Peter can't stand meeting new people. Matt loves and appreciates women. Peter thinks all women are "screwed up" and are all "manipulative liars". Matt currently has about eight women that are interested in him.

Peter has the big fat doughnut. Matt's doctor has told him he's as healthy as an ox while Peter's doctor is worried about his blood pressure, fat, weight, and overall health even though he's very young. When Matt hits an obstacle, he focuses his energy on how to solve it. When Peter hits an obstacle, he focuses his energy on why it happened to him and how unfair life is.

My advice to you is don't be a PETER. Become powerful by taking action.

Good luck!

P.S. If you have a success story or want to tell us what you thought of Element-X (the good, the bad, and the ugly), then shoot me an e-mail at:

bonnies@optonline.net

Please visit http://BonniesGang.com/

Next, Special Bonus Report - "Caveman Secrets"

A SIMPLE 5-STEP PLAN TO QUICKLY & EASILY UNLEASH YOUR HIDDEN SEXUAL POWERS AND CONFIDENCE

WARNING: Don't try __anything__ mentioned in this report unless you understand and fully-accept the concept of self-responsibility and understand and fully-accept that society, your parents, religion, the business-world, me __(especially me!)__, the Internet, etc., are not to blame if you screw up with this (or anything else, for that matter!) - __you are!__ This isn't medical advice! Always consult your Doctor

It never ceases to amaze me.

Having a healthy body is the **most basic requirement** for attracting the opposite sex. It's drummed into us all from childhood to stay fit and healthy... but it's absolutely astonishing how few men actually do look after themselves.

They puff-and-wheeze about with their beer-bellies wobbling like big fat marshmallows and expect women to fall at their feet!

Maybe its ignorance or maybe they're just plain lazy – the reasons don't matter; only the results - if you don't have even a basic standard of good health, you're putting yourself in an early grave... never mind **destroying** your ability to attract women!

There's <u>Nothing</u> More Sexy Than A Strong, Fit, Healthy Body!

There are just four **basic** things that determine how fit, strong, and healthy your body will be and they're all revealed right here in this **simple**, **no-nonsense**, **no-bull**, **rock-solid** report that you can understand, and use today.

It avoids the usual hyped up methods of increasing sexual health, power and ability and gives a laser-beam focus on what really matters.

It might be common sense, "everybody knows" kind of stuff. But it produces benefits - real permanent benefits that are hardly ever explained by anyone. These are infinitely superior to anything that can be brought on by drugs, medications, crackpot diets, and snake oil solutions!

All you have to do is actually apply it...

Discover The Outstanding "Secret" Benefits Of Actually Following Your Doctors Advice!

I'm sure your Doctor has often told you to eat more greens, get more exercise, blah, blah, blah...... and when you leave his office, you go for a big juicy hamburger, fries, and a shake!

If your Doctor ever actually bothered to tell you **why** you should do those things, you'd be both amazed at the fantastic benefits that will accrue to you and completely horrified at how your current lifestyle is depriving you of an incredible potential to be a dynamo of sexual health and power!

CAVEMAN SECRET #1: EAT RIGHT ... EAT RAW

The food you put into your mouth is the **biggest** factor in determining your sexual performance.

But don't worry! - I'm not going to complicate things with talk of calories and carbohydrates and all the other food-related things all the girls talk about but never **really** know what they mean.

I'm going to make it very simple and put it in Caveman language – in order to eat right, you need only understand the following statement:

The human body evolved over thousands of years, breathing, eating, and drinking what we found in nature as it is in nature today. Evolution designed our bodies to survive best on what food was available in nature –what was available was <u>fresh, raw, and unprepared</u>.

Not quite what you were expecting, was it?

Just think about it though – how long have humans cooked food and cultivated fields and processed TV-dinners and cooking recipes and all the things associated with modern eating habits? Maybe a few thousand years? (Actually, only a few decades if you're talking about TV-dinners!)

What did we eat for the thousands of years before that?

Exactly!... food that was fresh, raw, and unprepared. This is what made our bodies evolve and thrive!

Okay, if you have not rejected what I've just stated above in the same automatic way that many people respond to information that doesn't fit into their worldview, you're probably wondering what kind of diet plan or recommendations you should follow.

Eat 60% - 70% of your food fresh and raw.

I'm not saying you can't have a burger and fries every now and then.

This is simple, because you only have **two** things to do...

Cut – <u>Drastically</u>! – Your Consumption Of Cooked & Processed Food!

And just so you're clear: this includes refined **sugar**, **alcohol (in moderation alcohol is usually ok)**, **any kind of cooked or processed grains (bread, cereal or pasta)**.

And...

Eat As Much RAW Food As You Can!

This INCLUDES certified organic grass-fed meat and organic eggs and of course vegetables.

Many people who have switched to a mainly raw-food diet have reported some amazing benefits.

These include:

- **Less sweating, seborrhea, and greasy hair!**

- Some reversal of balding and hair loss

- **Minimal body odors (armpits, feet, genitals, etc.)!**

- Hands and feet no longer "**clammy**"!

- **No chilliness**, especially in the hands or feet!

- **Dramatic improvements in skin conditions!** Wrinkles and acne diminish, while corns, calluses, and other unsightly growths just fade away into oblivion.

- Excess fat melts away and muscles appear **well defined**!

- Better **able** to **withstand** long, drawn-out **exertion**, tendency to be **less** out of breath, and **better able to hold one's breath**.

- Less **n e r v o u s n e s s**, **s t r e s s**, **anxiety**, **irritability**, and even **shyness**!

- Improved concentration and memory, reflexes intuition and creativity.

Also, in keeping with the focus of this report, the following effects are also **readily** apparent:

- Sex drive goes **through the roof**!

- Iron-hard, long lasting erections (even for older men)

- Very **high quality** semen - an enormously high sperm count!

- Greatly increased **volume** of ejaculation (*Cum like a porn star*)!

All that from just following this advice – EAT MORE RAW FOOD.

In addition, most people start to see amazing results after as a little as 14 days.

If you want more information, there are **mountains** of **free** resources available all across the Web.

Start by checking out some of the following:

- http://RawPaleoDiet.org/ - **The Raw Paleolithic Diet Website**: a comprehensive resource of information, articles, and links on largely raw traditional diets that include raw animal products along with raw plant (vegetation) products.

- http://RawTimes.com/ - **The All Raw Times**: more information, articles, recipes, and contacts related to raw food diets.

- LivingNutrition.com - **Living Nutrition Magazine**: a premier health periodical, dedicated to teaching health seekers how to eat their natural diet of live raw fruits and vegetables, self-heal and build superb health the natural way.

There are many other sites too. Try using the search words "raw food diet" or something similar in your favorite search engine and see what you come up with!

Now, time to move on…

CAVEMAN SECRET #2: DRINK PLENTY OF PURE WATER

There is no roundabout way of putting this so I'll be perfectly blunt:

You Must Drink Lots Of

PURE Water __Every__ __Single__ __Day__
For The Rest Of Your Life!

Did you know that **more** than 75% of your body is <u>nothing but water</u>?

It's true.

That's why water is so important – it is **directly** involved in most, if not all, of the activities that your body performs to stay healthy and alive.

You probably wouldn't live much more than 10 days without it. To maintain good health, you must drink at least **eight** glasses of pure water **every day!**

Notice how I'm saying **<u>pure</u>** water? Back in the caveman day, that's all they had - no pollution, no additives … nothing but pure water.

Any old water will keep you alive as long as it is reasonably free of contamination and micro-organism. To see real benefits, drink PURE filtered water

Have you ever seen those bottled waters that say, "Drink this because it has lots of minerals in it!"?

Avoid them!

Does your tap-water have fluoride and chlorine and God-only-knows-what in it?

Avoid unfiltered tap water too, if you can!

Why is it so important that the water you drink be pure?

Well, some people hold belief that the essential minerals their body needs are derived from the water they drink. While it is true that you do need minerals, the source for these minerals are in the **food you eat** – *__not in the water you drink!__*

Your body is able to use few, if any, of the minerals dissolved in water. These minerals could actually **hinder** water from carrying out its natural functions of keeping your body chemistry **regulated** and **functioning** properly.

Of all the various types of water such as rain, snow-melt, hard, soft, de-ionized, boiled, and distilled – __only pure spring water and filtered water are good for your body.__

As a result, spring or filtered water has:

- no **taste**.
- no **color**.
- no **odor.**
- no **bacteria**.
- no **heavy metals**.
- no **acids**.
- no **organic materials**.
- no **toxic chemicals**.
- no **poisons**.

Filtered water enters your body clean and pure and free to absorb and wash away accumulated poisons and toxins and carry out its other vital functions.

You Can filter Water Yourself With A Low-Cost Home filter!

If you go to any place that sells household appliances, you should find a variety of home water filters available. *But be warned!* – prices can vary considerably and <u>you do get what you pay for</u> in terms of reliability and life-span. Buy the best quality you can afford.

I promise you won't regret it one bit!

Here's why...

People who regularly drink a lot of pure water

have reported:

- All those annoying aches and pain - simply disappear– <u>without</u> drugs, homeopathy or meditation!

- Excess weight **disappears**
-
- Skin becomes soft and subtle

- **"Crows-feet" disappear from the face!**

You'll notice than some of the above tie-in with reported results in the diet section above. I have personally found that **combining** the two produces much more **dramatic** results that just changing your diet or just drinking pure water. Now, you might be thinking: "*This is all great for my general **health**, but what is it going to do for my **sex life and confidence** !?*"

Okay, well... remember the benefits achieved with the change of diet mentioned in the above section and in Element-X? (**Increased** sex drive, **stronger** and **longer lasting** erections, and much **improved quality**, **volume**, and **flavor** of semen.)

They increase even more!

That's right; you'll experience a **m a s s i v e** acceleration of these effects.

Take this rather silly analogy:

Right now, think of yourself as being a little airplane chugging along with a propeller. Changing your diet as described in the previous section is like adding a jet engine.

But using pure water too is like turning on the afterburners!

Whoooooooooooooooooosh!!!

CAVEMAN SECRET #3: GET ENOUGH EXERCISE

This section is simple indeed. You probably already have heard this information a hundred times, but always ignore it. Now that you have made the commitment to improve yourself (and get laid more) now is the time to heed this advise.

If you are trying to make yourself attractive to the opposite sex (and keep your health while you're at it!), you **must** spend time exercising your body to keep it in shape.

You Can't Expect to Attract Desirable women If You're A Big Fatty Who Sits On Your Ass All Day Watching TV!

Don't bother with gyms and aerobics classes if you can't afford it. You probably won't stick with them anyway, so you'll just be wasting your time and money.

Becoming and staying fit should not be an expensive chore.

All you have to do is spend time a few days each week doing some physical activity, you enjoy.

It could be as simple as working in the yard or around the house.

Or going swimming.

Or, better still, joining a dance class (Women love men who can dance properly!)

It really doesn't matter what activity you choose to do. The point is: **Get out there and do something – anything.**

Get up off your ass and just do it!

No excuses, no ifs-and-buts, - just lift yourself out of your chair and do something – *d o anything!*

Time to move on …

CAVEMAN SECRET #4: SLEEEEEEEEP!

This one really is a no-brainer.

If you're one of those people who thinks it's a good idea to go to work all day and then stay out partying all night with only an hour or two of sleep in between, then you need to pay close attention to this:

Get more sleep!

Sleep allows your body and mind to rest and repair after the day. Simple as that! If you're not getting enough of it, you're storing up trouble.

I recommend that you have eight hours of sleep a night. I know that's not going to happen because you are busy with smokin' hot women – but do your best.

This may not be necessary!

Getting fewer hours of better quality sleep is more beneficial than 8 hours of poor disturbed sleep.

For a variety of reasons, you might not be able to stick to a rigid sleep schedule but, for your own sake, do try!

Enough said!

CAVEMAN SECRET #5
HOW ONE SIMPLE ACTION CAN IMPROVE
YOUR LIFE MORE THAN ANYTHING ELSE!

A caveman walked every day --- so should you.

These simple directions contain an extraordinary psychological secret and energy boost that contributed to my - and many other peoples' - success.

Here it is…

There is one single thing that you can do, starting tomorrow, to improve your life, sex life and confidence more than anything else.

It's not difficult to remember.

It's not difficult to do.

It doesn't require any special clothing.

It doesn't require any special equipment.

Here it is...

As Soon As You Wake Up In The Morning... Get Yourself Out Of Your House!

When you first open your eyes, you'll probably then want to use the bathroom, brush your teeth and use a warm wash-cloth to scrub the sleep out of your face.

Dress yourself. Drink a glass of water. Put on a pair of walking shoes. Get out the door.

Look at your watch and note the time.

Now ...Start walking, and after twenty minutes, turn around and start walking home.

That's it.

Do this every day, whether you're at home or away.

When you get back home, shower, shave, and put on some fresh clothes.

This is the way you start your day before you start your day.

Do it <u>every day</u> for the rest of your life.

This caveman simple daily activity will change your physical and mental being for the better.

Always the simple stuff **really** changes you.

I don't exactly know why... but... **I guarantee it to be true!**

Arguably, the greatest discovery of this century was that of Einstein's Theory of Relativity ... $E = mc^2$.

How much are those simple letters "$E = mc^2$" worth?

Although they only take up perhaps one inch of space on one line of paper, those simple letters are worth untold <u>trillions</u> of dollars.

If you come across a safe which has ten million dollars locked inside of it... and... you are told a simple 10-digit combination is necessary to open that safe... how valuable to you are those simple ten digits?

My point: Many people judge the worth or the value of information by the volume or the weight of the information.

Many people think a 300-page hard cover book filled with nothing but gibberish is worth many times more than a 2-page PDF report filled with hard-hitting advice; advice so valuable, it literally changes their lives.

Or a few paragraphs, for that matter…

The "presentation" of the information doesn't matter… the information itself is what is vital. Stripped down of all the mumbo-jumbo, you've got it now. You've got "the cavemen secrets" for building your confidence and boosting your sexual powers.

If you haven't already, finish part one and two of this book and go out there and make me proud.

http://BonniesGang.com

www.ingramcontent.com/pod-product-compliance
Lightning Source LLC
Chambersburg PA
CBHW031510270326
41930CB00006B/347